D1269316

615.9
H
Hyams
Poisons

87-1857

JUN 1987

FLESH PUBLIC LIBRARY
PIQUA, OHIO

DISCARD

Poisons

Jay Hyams

FLESH PUBLIC LIBRARY

American Family Health Institute™

Medical Board

Stanley J. Dudrick, MD
Clinical Professor of Surgery
University of Texas Medical School, Houston, Texas

Jo Eland, RN, PhD
Assistant Professor, University of Iowa
Iowa City, Iowa

Dennis E. Leavelle, MD
Consulting Pathologist, Department of Laboratory Medicine
Mayo Clinic, Rochester, Minnesota

Julena Lind, MN, RN
Director of Education, Center for Health Information, Education and Research
at California Medical Center, Los Angeles, California

Ara G. Paul, PhD
Dean, College of Pharmacy, University of Michigan
Ann Arbor, Michigan

Richard Payne, MD
Clinical Assistant Neurologist, Memorial Sloan-Kettering Cancer Center
New York, New York

William R. Truscott, MD
Diplomate, American Academy of Family Practice, Lansdale Medical Group
Lansdale, Pennsylvania

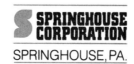

SPRINGHOUSE CORPORATION
SPRINGHOUSE, PA.

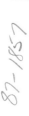

87-1857

Program Director
Stanley Loeb

Clinical Director
Barbara McVan, RN

Clinical Editor
Donna Hilton, RN,
CCRN, CEN

Art Director
John Hubbard

Designer
Lorraine Lostracco
Carbo

**Editorial Services
Supervisor**
David Moreau

Production Manager
Wilbur Davidson

The charter of the American Family Health Institute is to research and produce high-quality publications that enhance the health of individuals and their families. Essential to health are physical, emotional, and social well-being, not just the absence of illness or infirmity. The Institute's Medical Board has produced the *Health and Fitness* books to share up-to-date and authoritative information that can give readers greater personal control over their health maintenance.

© 1986 by Springhouse Corporation,
1111 Bethlehem Pike, Springhouse,
Pa. 19477

All rights reserved. Reproduction in
whole or part by any means whatso-
ever without written permission of
the publisher is prohibited by law.
Printed in the United States of America.

Library of Congress Cataloging-in-
Publication Data
Hyams, Jay, 1949-
　　Poisons.
　　Includes index.
　　1. Toxicology—Popular works.　　2.
Poisons—Safety measures—Popular works.
　　3. Toxicological emergencies—Popular
works.　　4. Consumer education. I. Brunner,
Lillian Sholtis.　　II. American Family Health
Institute. Medical Board. III. Title. IV. Series.
　　[DNLM: 1. Toxicology—popular works.
QV 600 H992p]
RA1213.H93　　1986　　615.9'
85-27934
ISBN 0-87434-027-6

The procedures and explanations given in this publication are based on research and consultation with medical and nursing authorities. To the best of our knowledge, these procedures and explanations reflect currently accepted medical practice; never-theless, they can't be considered absolute and universal recommendations. For indi-vidual application, treatment suggestions must be considered in light of the individual's health, subject to a doctor's specific recommendations. The authors and the publisher disclaim responsibility for any adverse effects resulting directly or indi-rectly from the suggested procedures, from any undetected errors, or from the read-er's misunderstanding of the text.

Contents

Poisons

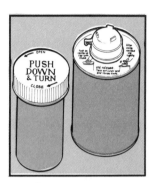

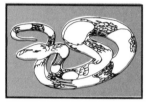

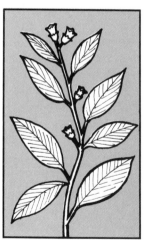

87-185> JUN 1987

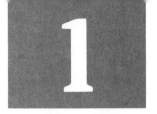

The Poisons in Our World

Love potions and poison arrows

When a bartender invites you to "name your poison," he's making a nice play on words. A poison, in the original sense of the word, is something to drink (the word poison *is a close relative of the words* potable *and* potion: *they come from a Latin word meaning "a drink"). The meaning of* poison *changed from "a drink" to "a deadly drink" during the Middle Ages, when various chemicals were frequently added to drinks. Some of these "doctored" beverages were made to kill, but most were "love potions," special brews meant to make people fall in love. They must not have worked too well— or perhaps they had bad side effects—for* poison *came to have the deadly significance it has today.*

Further proof that love potions didn't work well is supplied by the word venom, *which we use for the poisonous substances produced by certain animals and insects.* Venom *comes from* venin—*a word related to Venus, goddess of love, that was also originally used for love potions.*

If something's poisonous, it's toxic. Toxic *comes from a word meaning "poison for arrows." The related word* toxin *refers to the poisons found in certain plants, bacteria, and venoms.*

Some poisons come in little glass bottles embossed with a skull and crossbones. Some come in big steel cans marked, "Danger: Harmful if swallowed." Some poisons come from the fangs of snakes and the stingers of bees. There are poisons that make newspaper headlines: industrial wastes that pollute rivers and chemical gases that foul the air. We hear about some poisons quite frequently: food poisoning, lead poisoning, carbon monoxide poisoning. And we've all seen exciting films about heroic adventurers in faraway lands faced with angry natives armed with poison-tipped arrows.

Unfortunately, many poisons come in attractive, familiar wrappers and can be found on the shelves of your own home: aspirin and ammonia, cleaning fluids and cold medicines, drain cleaners and oven cleaners, paints and perfumes—the list of the poisons we live with goes on and on.

You probably don't think of such everyday things as poisonous. After all, cleaning fluids, cold medicines, and perfumes aren't like snake venom or the sticky goo into which a native dips his arrow: they aren't made to do harm, but to help keep us clean, healthy, and happy. They play important roles in our lives, and few of us would like to do without them. But there's another, ever-present side to these everyday household products—because of the chemicals they contain, they're potential poisons.

Poisons cause injury chemically

In the broadest sense, a poison is anything that chemically causes illness or death if it gets into or onto a human body in sufficient quantity. The word *chemically* is important: a bullet shot into you will cause illness or death, but it does so by piercing and disrupting your vital organs. A poison causes injury chemically: it either changes the way your body works—makes your heart beat too fast, for example— or reacts with your body's tissue—as when an acid burns your skin.

"Sufficient quantity" is important, too: some substances are harmful in tiny amounts; some are harmful only in relatively large amounts. You're probably

Not how much but with what
Some substances become harmful when taken in combination with another substance: the combination of alcohol and Valium, for example, can be extremely dangerous.

Drugs as poisons
All prescription and non-prescription drugs are potential poisons: they're created to affect us chemically. In correct doses, they keep us well or treat illnesses; in incorrect doses, they can cause harm. Medicinal drugs are closely related to poisons; see page 10.

How many poisonous substances are there?
Approximately 4 million natural and synthetic substances have been identified, and the number is growing every year because of new chemicals created by industry. However, fewer than 3,000 of these substances are responsible for accidental poisonings.

familiar with the names of some of the substances that are harmful in tiny amounts. Cyanide and strychnine are examples—as little as a drop of either one is enough to kill an adult. Such substances are what we usually think of as poisons.

They aren't the only poisons in our world, however. Any substance that can affect you chemically has the potential to harm you if it gets into or onto your body in sufficient quantity. However, with some substances, the amount necessary to cause harm (sometimes called the toxic dose) is so large that the substances are considered nontoxic. Unfortunately, the number of nontoxic substances is small compared to the number of potentially poisonous substances.

Poisonous substances
What kinds of substances cause injury chemically? Poisons come in many forms—liquids, gases, solids—and come from many sources. They can be either natural or synthetic (created in a laboratory).

Natural poisons include the toxic chemicals present in many different kinds of plants and the venoms produced by various animals, such as snakes and spiders. Other natural poisons are the toxic substances produced by various bacteria in food.

Synthetic poisons include industrial chemicals and minerals, the chemicals used in household products, and all prescription and nonprescription drugs.

The poisons around us
Poisons are all around us. You can decide to avoid some of them, of course. If you never go outside (and don't keep strange pets), you may never encounter a poisonous snake, but you can't avoid encountering all the poisons in our world. Your job may require you to come in contact with dangerous chemicals; you certainly make use of potentially dangerous chemicals at home.

With the exception of the substances we use as poisons—to kill weeds, bugs, and rats, for instance—the poisons in our world appear under other names, names that reflect the ways we use them. We call them detergents, drain cleaners, cold medicines, nail polish remover. We rarely call them by their chemical names—names that might suggest their potential for causing harm. And used properly, these potential poisons are safe; but they can all become dangerous poisons if they're misused; abused; or if they enter or touch our bodies in sufficient amounts. Such events

The size and health of the victim
Because of their small size, children are more vulnerable to smaller doses of poisons than are adults. The elderly and infirm are more likely to be hurt by some poisons, such as food poisons, than younger or healthier people.

A single exposure
Although they usually involve repeated exposures to small doses of a poison, chronic poisonings can result from a single exposure that doesn't cause an immediate reaction but causes disease years later. Examples are exposure to radioactive elements or carcinogens (cancer-causing substances).

are called poisonings.

Acute poisonings

There are two kinds of poisoning: acute poisoning and chronic poisoning. Acute poisonings are usually the result of an accidental poisoning or a suicide attempt.

An acute poisoning is a sudden poisoning: the effects of the poison on the body are immediate or occur shortly after the exposure. The symptoms run a short course and can be mild or severe, depending on several factors, including the type of poison, the amount involved, the way the poison enters the body, the length of time it stays in the body, and the age, size, and health of the victim.

Chronic poisonings

Chronic poisonings usually involve repeated exposures to small doses of a poison. Symptoms may take months or years to develop, and identification of the cause of such a poisoning may be extremely difficult—if it's even recognized as a poisoning.

Chronic poisonings are usually the result of repeated exposures to toxic substances in the workplace or the environment. For example, lead poisoning in children—caused by the ingestion of pieces of lead-based paint over a period of time—is a form of chronic poisoning.

The effects of poisons

Once in or on the victim's body, poisons cause damage in various ways. The damage can be divided into two categories: local effects and systemic effects.

Local effects occur at the place where the poison entered or touched the body. An acid, for example, burns any skin or tissue (such as the lining of the mouth) it touches.

Systemic effects involve the victim's central nervous system, breathing, blood circulation, or vital organs (particularly the liver, kidneys, and lungs). Systemic effects result when a poison is absorbed into the blood and carried through the body. Systemic effects are more serious than local effects; they can be life-threatening.

Many poisons can cause both local and systemic effects—they cause damage entering the body and further damage once inside. Although most poisons affect several parts of the body, serious illness or death usually results from damage to one organ (such as the liver) or body function (such as breathing or

The liver and kidneys
The liver and kidneys work to keep blood free of toxic substances; in an accidental poisoning, toxic substances can overtax these organs and interfere with their proper function.

How poisons enter our bodies
Poisons can enter our bodies in four ways:

1. Ingestion (by mouth)
Nearly 90% of all poisoning accidents involve ingested, or swallowed, poisons.

2. Inhalation (by nose or mouth)
Many kinds of inhaled gases, fumes, vapors, and dusts can cause injury. Some of these (such as carbon monoxide) cause acute poisonings; some (such as asbestos dust) cause chronic poisonings.

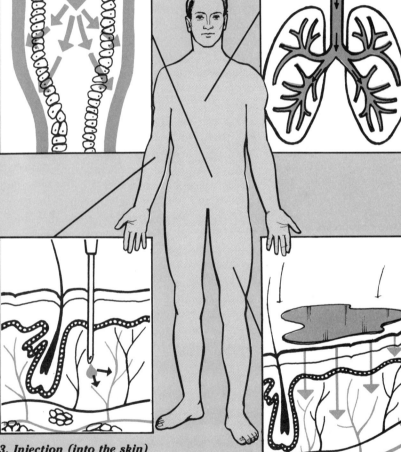

3. Injection (into the skin)
Doctors and nurses use hypodermic needles to inject medicinal drugs into our bodies. Snakes and insects inject poisons into our bodies when they bite or sting: the poison enters the skin through the snake's fangs or the insect's stinger. Many drug overdoses (intentional or accidental) involve injected poisons.

4. Absorption (through the skin or into the eyes)
A variety of substances cause damage when they come in contact with the skin or the eyes. Many of these substances can cause further damage if they're absorbed through the skin into the blood.

blood circulation).

First-aid principles for poisonings

The longer a poison stays in or on your body, the more damage it does. All poisonings are therefore medical emergencies and require immediate attention.

The damage caused by a poison is in large part determined by how the poison enters the body, and first-aid measures differ according to the route of entry.

Ingested poisons

Ingested poisons are divided into three general categories:
• Substances that are neither corrosive (caustic) nor petroleum-like: this category includes most medicines and drugs, plants, food poisoning, and many household products.
• Corrosive (caustic) substances: this category includes household bleaches, metal polishes, antirust solutions, paint and varnish removers, drain cleaners, refrigerants, fertilizers, and photographic developers.
• Petroleum-like substances: this category includes floor polish and wax, furniture polish and wax, gasoline, kerosene, and lighter fluid.

Most accidental ingested poisonings involve substances that are neither corrosive nor petroleum-like. The variety of these substances is enormous and isn't restricted to liquids. With some substances (such as plants that irritate the skin), there may be local effects, but the main concern following the ingestion of any substance is the possibility of systemic effects.

First aid for ingested noncorrosive and non–petroleum-like substances is directed at getting the poison out of the body, which is best accomplished by making the victim vomit. As we'll see (page 40), the best way to induce vomiting is with ipecac syrup.

Corrosives burn or destroy tissue through their chemical action. Swallowing a corrosive substance, such as an acid or an alkali, will cause immediate local effects. These poisons burn skin: they burn the lips and skin around the victim's mouth and burn the lining of the victim's mouth, throat, and stomach. Absorbed into the blood, they can cause systemic effects: acids, for example, can cause hemorrhages; alkalis can cause difficult breathing.

The victim of an ingested corrosive substance requires immediate medical care. First aid for this kind

Swallowing rattlesnake venom
The way a poisonous substance enters your body can determine whether or not the substance harms you. Rattlesnake venom injected into your blood (as can happen when a rattlesnake bites you) is dangerous; the same venom can be swallowed with no harmful results. This is because the venom is composed of proteins, and the digestive actions of your stomach break up the proteins, making them harmless. Insoluble substances—substances that can't be dissolved in a liquid and therefore can't get into your bloodstream—may pass through your body (and be lost in the feces) virtually unchanged. The elemental mercury in a thermometer is an example of this kind of insoluble substance.

of poisoning depends on what was ingested, but one rule applies to all corrosives—don't make the victim vomit. Should the victim vomit the corrosive, it will again burn the sensitive lining of the throat and mouth. In some cases, demulcents (soothing substances) such as milk, egg white, aluminum hydroxide gel, gelatin solution, flour and water, or vegetable oil may dilute the corrosive, but these should be given to the victim only if so directed by a poison control center, doctor, or hospital emergency room.

Similarly, the victim of an ingested petroleum-like substance should not be made to vomit. Petroleum-like products give off fumes that can cause a severe type of pneumonia, and these fumes may be inhaled into the lungs during vomiting.

First-aid measures
Specific guidance for the first-aid treatment of poisonings is given in Chapter 6, beginning on page 39.

Inhaled poisons

Inhaling certain gases, vapors, fumes, and dusts may cause only irritation to the body's respiratory tract: nose, mouth, windpipe, and lungs. Some of these poisons, however, cause systemic effects when they're absorbed from the lungs into the blood. Carbon monoxide gas, for example, has an effect on blood that prevents it from carrying oxygen.

The basic first-aid procedure for an inhaled poison is to get the victim to fresh air immediately. Artificial respiration may then be necessary.

Injected poisons

Most injected poisons produce immediate local effects: pain, tenderness, and swelling at the site of the injection. Systemic effects take longer to develop and depend on the amount of the poison that enters the blood.

The local effects of an injected poison can be treated with first-aid measures (putting meat tenderizer on a bee sting, for example); treatment of systemic effects, however, requires expert medical attention. There's no way to get the poison out (sucking out snake venom is no longer recommended).

Poisons and time
It takes time for systemic effects to occur—the poison must be absorbed into the blood. Thus, all first-aid measures for poisoning accidents stress speed: the sooner the poison is removed from the body or its action somehow nullified, the less damage the poison will cause.

Absorbed poisons

Absorbed poisons—those that come in contact with the skin—usually cause immediate local effects. Acids, for example, burn the skin. Some chemicals, such as those found in certain insecticides, are rapidly absorbed into the bloodstream through the skin; once in the blood, they can cause systemic effects.

First aid for absorbed poisons is directed at getting the poison off the skin and diluting it.

All substances are poisons

The close relationship between poisons and medicinal drugs has been noted by medical writers throughout history. The 16th-century Swiss physician Paracelsus wrote, "All substances are poisons; there is none that is not a poison. The right dose differentiates a poison and a remedy." Claude Bernard, the 19th-century French physiologist known as the father of experimental medicine, wrote, "Poisons can be employed as agents of life's destruction or as means for the relief of disease."

Aspirin as poison

The chemical in aspirin has an effect on the body's central nervous system. In proper doses, the chemical lessens sensitivity to pain. In excessive doses, this same painkilling chemical prevents the central nervous system from working properly: breathing becomes difficult, the heart and other organs are affected—and death may occur.

Willow tree bark

The history of aspirin goes back to a plant—the willow tree. In ancient times, people boiled the bark of willow trees to make an anti-fever medicine. Modern chemists isolated the bark's active ingredient and named it salicylate, from the Latin salix ("willow").

Poisons and medicinal drugs

Medicinal drugs are the easiest to identify of the potential poisons in our world. In a sense, medicinal drugs are "beneficial poisons." Indeed, the history of medicinal drugs is tied to the history of poisons. Understanding some of that history will help you understand where poisons come from and how they work.

Certain chemicals can be either harmful—poisonous—or helpful—medicinal—depending on the amount. Like poisons, medicinal drugs either change the way your body works or react with your body's tissue. Poisons cause harmful changes or reactions; medicinal drugs cause beneficial changes or reactions. The difference between being hurt or helped by any particular chemical substance is frequently in the dosage, the amount taken into the body.

For example, two aspirin tablets, swallowed with some water, will relieve a headache; an overdose of aspirin—an amount greater than the prescribed dose—can cause serious stomach upset, nausea, rapid breathing, and vomiting. In excessive doses, aspirin can be fatal. Thus, one of the most useful medicinal drugs in our world becomes a dangerous poison when too much is taken.

Deadly plants

The close relationship between the chemicals used in poisons and those used in medicinal drugs reflects their common origin: many come from plants.

Humans have been making use of the active ingredients—the chemicals—found in plants since earliest times. Our prehistoric ancestors discovered these plant chemicals through painful firsthand experience—they learned that some plants were harmless if eaten and could be used as food and other plants caused illness or death if eaten. These deadly plants fascinated early humans: the history of both poisons and modern medicine begins with that fascination.

The active ingredients in plants haven't changed with time, but our ability to make use of them has. We've learned how to isolate the active ingredients in plants and synthesize our own products chemically—we can combine plants' natural chemicals to create new, complex chemicals. By understanding the chemicals' effects, we can design particular medicinal drugs to combat particular diseases.

Poisons that heal

Many plant chemicals once used to make poisons are now used to make medicinal drugs. The following are only a few examples:

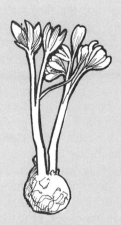

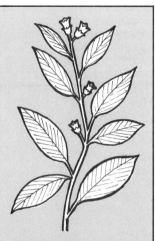

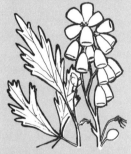

Aconite

"Here's to my love," toasts the heartbroken Romeo, downing a cup of poison. He dies with dramatic speed and falls near the body of his beloved Juliet. Shakespearean scholars agree that the poison in Romeo's cup was aconite. Aconite is obtained from a plant known as Aconitum napellus. This plant is also known as monkshood, because its flowers look like a monk's hood, and wolfsbane, because old superstitions held it was useful in warding off werewolves. Aconite is still with us, but it's no longer used only as a poison; instead, it has been used as a sedative and as an ointment to relieve the pain of rheumatism.

Henbane

Hamlet must face the fact that his father was murdered with "cursed hebenon." Today, we know hebenon as henbane. It's obtained from a plant called Hyoscyamus niger and is used medicinally as a muscle relaxant.

Colchicine

An extract of the autumn crocus (Colchicum autumnale), colchicine is used in treating cancer, gout, and arthritis; the ancient Romans used it as a poison.

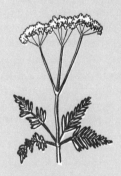

Coniine

Poison hemlock was the "state poison" of ancient Athens, used to execute criminals and other unwanted persons. Its most famous victim was the philosopher Socrates, condemned to drink a cup of hemlock for "corrupting the youth of Athens." Today, the active ingredient of poison hemlock, coniine, serves as a sedative, painkiller, and antispasmodic (drug that prevents or relieves muscle spasms or convulsions).

Belladonna

Medieval witches claimed they had visions of the devil when they ate belladonna. This plant (Atropa belladonna) was also part of the special witches' brew that supposedly made broomsticks fly. Today, belladonna is an important medicinal drug, used in many ways, including the treatment of ulcers and stomach spasms.

Curare

Perhaps the best example of a poison that has become an important medicine is curare. One of the deadliest poisons known, curare is used by South American Indians as an arrow poison; they make it from a substance found in local trees. Curare kills by quickly relaxing all the victim's muscles. Within seconds, this relaxation becomes paralysis, and the victim stops breathing. Laboratory-made curare drugs are used today in most hospitals. Tiny amounts are used during surgery to relax the patient's muscles, making operations easier and safer.

Antidotes

Antidotes are substances that either prevent a poison from being absorbed or prevent it from causing damage once it is absorbed. For example, a drug known as acetylcysteine has proven effective as an antidote to acetaminophen poisoning (acetaminophen is an aspirin substitute used in such products as Tylenol, Datril, and Anacin 3). Unfortunately, specific antidotes exist for less than 2% of all poisons.

Antidotes are sometimes included on the labels of product containers. Pay no attention to such information. It may be either inaccurate or out of date.

The best-known antidotes are those used to counteract snake venoms. Antidotes are produced by inoculating an animal, usually a horse, with small doses of snake venom. The horse gradually builds up a resistance to the venom in its blood. Blood serum (the liquid part of blood) taken from immunized horses can be injected into snakebite victims. Such an "antivenom" serum is known as an antivenin. (One drawback to this kind of antidote is that some people are allergic to horse serum.)

The active ingredients found in plants are a major source of the chemicals used in both medicinal drugs and poisons. The poisonous substances present in certain animals—such as snakes and spiders—are other sources. Our ancient ancestors used these poisons to kill their enemies; modern medical researchers use them to keep people well or heal the sick.

Poisons and medicines have also been produced from the minerals present in the earth. For example, sulfur (the "brimstone" of the Bible) is used as an insecticide and in the treatment of skin diseases. Chlorine in one form gives us DDT; in another, it produces the anesthetic chloroform. Even arsenic, a popular poison for many centuries, has seen medicinal uses; one of its compounds is used to make Salvarsan, formerly used in the treatment of venereal diseases.

Plants and animals still provide the chemicals used in many drugs, but modern manufacturers usually prefer to create their own chemicals, which are purer and more uniform than natural chemicals. Today, most prescription drugs are made of chemicals created in a laboratory. These are wonderful medicines, and they have changed our world. Dramatic advances in the field of medicine made during the 1950s brought us protection against ailments that were once fatal or disabling. Polio is only one example. These same advances have also left us surrounded by medicines—all of which are potential poisons, and some of which once were poisons.

2

Poison Prevention

Proof of progress
Between 1973 and 1982 there was a 46% decrease in children's hospital visits for ingestion of prescription drugs, and deaths among children under age 5 due to all household products dropped 75% between 1972 and 1981.

Statistics tell us this:

- Nearly 2 million Americans are poisoned each year.
- Most poisonings (more than 90%) are accidental.
- Most poisonings (more than 90%) occur in the victim's home.
- Most victims of accidental poisonings (nearly 70%) are between the ages of 1 and 5.
- Over 80% of poisonings involve ingested, or swallowed, poisons.
- The majority of poisonings (92%) involve a single substance.

All those numbers add up to two important facts: accidental poisonings occur at home, and most accidental poisonings involve children. The good news is that few accidental poisonings are fatal. What's more, accidental poisonings can be prevented. Doing so means keeping children and poisons apart and handling dangerous substances, including medicines, properly.

What's being done

Accidental poisonings can be prevented—and are being prevented. The number of poisonings among children and the number of deaths from accidental poisonings have fallen dramatically over the past few years. Among the factors responsible for this are the childproof closures used on many products and the efforts of our nation's poison control centers.

Progress is being made, but tens of thousands of children each year still suffer from contact with hazardous substances, and many of them die. Many adults, too, fall victim to accidental poisonings.

Childproof caps and poison control centers exist for your protection. Recognizing the importance of these efforts—and making use of them—is the beginning of poison prevention.

Poison prevention packaging

It isn't always easy to open a bottle of aspirin these days. You have to look at the cap, twist it around a bit, and then pry it off. All this looking and twisting may result in some slight inconvenience, but before you lose your temper with one of these tops, remem-

How hard is too hard?

Poison prevention packaging is a compromise between opening ease for adults and difficult access for children. If the tops were so difficult that no children could open them, many adults wouldn't be able to open the packages either.

ber that they're designed to save children's lives.

And they work. During the 1940s, about 140 children died each year from overdoses of aspirin; that number is now down to 10 to 25, and it goes down more each year.

Safety tops (also called childproof caps or child-resistant tops) are the result of the Poison Prevention Packaging Act of 1970, administered by the U.S. Consumer Products Safety Commission. This act requires that certain household products found to be hazardous or potentially hazardous must be sold in safety packaging that most children under age 5 can't open.

According to the Poison Prevention Packaging Act, child-resistant tops must be sufficiently difficult to open so that they can't be opened by 80% of children under age 5. At the same time, these tops must be easy enough to open so that 90% of adults can open and close them without trouble.

Poison control centers

Poison control centers are located all across the coun-

Safety closure: A must

Drugs currently required to be in safety packaging:

- *prescription drugs in oral dosage form*
- *all controlled drugs in oral dosage form*
- *aspirin products, except for certain effervescent and powder forms*
- *oil of wintergreen (methyl salicylate)*
- *preparations containing iron, including dietary supplements*
- *acetaminophen products (aspirin substitutes).*

Several other products are available in safety packaging. These include:
- *certain furniture polishes*
- *products containing potassium and sodium hydroxide or both (certain oven and drain cleaners)*
- *turpentine*
- *kindling and illuminating fluids, such as cigarette*

and charcoal lighter fluids
- *sulfuric acid*
- *antifreeze (ethylene glycol)*
- *windshield washer solution (methyl alcohol)*
- *paint solvents.*

Exceptions

Some people, including the elderly and those with handicaps like arthritis, can't open safety tops. The law allows two ways for these people to get conventional packages:

- *Manufacturers are permitted to market one size of a product in conventional packaging if the same product is also available in child-resistant packaging. However, the conventional packaging must have a label that clearly states:* This package for households without young children *or, if the package is very small:* Package not child-

resistant
- *The consumer can request that prescription medicines be put into conventional packages without safety closures. Although some pharmacists may ask for a written statement from a purchaser before providing a conventional closure, this isn't a requirement of the law.*

Childproof tops aren't enough to prevent accidental poisonings: in homes where there are children, all potential poisons, regardless of closure, must be kept out of sight and out of reach of children.

Childproof closures save children's lives—use them. Ask your pharmacist to provide safety closures on all medicine containers, and use household products that are available in childproof packages. Refasten safety closures immediately after use.

Telephone stickers

Many poison control centers distribute telephone stickers with the center's phone number. These stickers are of enormous value—you should have one stuck on or near every phone in your home.

Memory buttons

Some phones now have memory buttons; you may want to assign one of these buttons to the poison control center's number.

try. Many are part of a nationwide organization called the American Association of Poison Control Centers.

The main purpose of poison control centers is to provide emergency help to poison victims and doctors treating poison victims. Most requests for help come by phone. Each poison control center has access to up-to-date information provided by several data-collection programs. Within minutes, the poison control center staff can recommend the proper treatment.

Poison control centers have proved to be an effective system for aiding poison victims. They're responsible in large part for the dramatic decline in the number of poison-related deaths.

They're also responsible for the greater public awareness of the dangers of poisoning. Educating the public, particularly parents, about how to prevent accidental poisonings is one of the tasks of poison control centers.

No matter where you live, there's a poison control center near you. You can find its phone number in

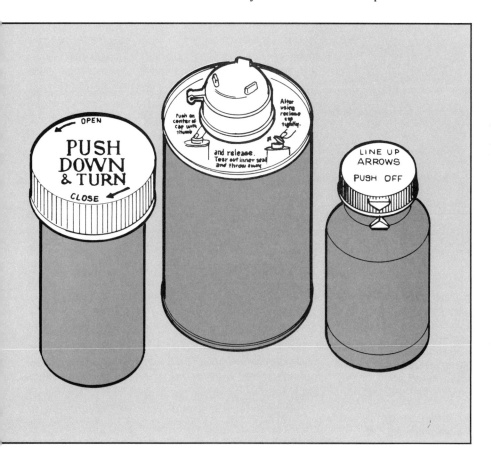

Grandmother's purse
*Many poisonings occur
when a child visits grand-
parents and goes through
the medicine cabinet or
grandmother's purse. If you
or others in your family
must use conventional
packaging, you'll have to
be especially alert.*

your telephone directory. This number should be on or near every telephone in your home. In the event of a poisoning or suspected poisoning, call the poison control center. (See page 39 for specific information on contacting poison control centers in the event of an emergency.)

What you can do

The most important factor in poison prevention is how you deal with the poisons in your home. This means handling medicines properly, using household products safely and in the manner in which they were made to be used, keeping all household products and medicines in their original containers, and keeping all hazardous substances out of the sight and reach of children.

The remainder of this book is devoted to those topics, but you can find smaller, abbreviated versions of these same topics all around your house: they're on the labels of most of the medicines and products you use.

Labels

Your doctor can't pay you a house call each time you have to take a prescribed medicine, and the manufacturers of household products can't stop by each time you reach for one of their products. Even so, you're not completely on your own when you take medicine or use a household product—you have the label to guide you.

Read labels. Read the label before you buy any household product. Make sure you know what the product is made to do and make sure you understand how it should be used. In particular, make sure you'll be able to use the product safely. Read the safety precautions—if the product seems dangerous, see if you can find another that will do the same job but is less dangerous. Buy amounts you can use; don't buy large containers that you'll have to store. And read the label again—including the safety precautions—each time you use the product.

**Safety closures don't
last forever**
*Safety closures lose their ef-
fectiveness through re-
peated use, so new
packaging must be used
when prescriptions are refilled. In the case of glass
containers, using new caps
for refills is enough to meet
the law's requirements.*

Read the labels of all prescription medicines before you leave the pharmacy. Make sure the medicine is what the doctor prescribed and that you understand how it's meant to be taken. And read the label again each time you use the medicine.

Follow all label instructions. In particular, remember to "use only as directed" and "keep out of the reach of children."

3

Poison-Proofing Your Home

Don't poison the environment
You can safely dispose of most medicines and drugs by flushing them down a toilet or pouring them down a sink. Check the label first, however, for any special instructions. (Rinse out the container and dispose of it where children can't get at it.) Throwing away household products, automotive supplies, pesticides, or other chemicals is another matter. If you pour them down the sink or into the ground, they'll pollute our environment. The best way to get rid of such chemicals is to use them for their intended purpose. If that isn't possible, store them safely. If you have products that might be useful to someone else—such as leftover paint—donate them to a charitable organization. Be especially careful with dangerous chemicals like pesticides. Follow the label directions for proper disposal. Never dump such products in the trash. If you have any doubts, call your local or state waste management agency.

You can't throw out every poison and potential poison in your home. To do so would mean going without medicines, detergents, cleansers, paints, polishes—it would mean going without most of the products you depend on every day to make your life healthy and enjoyable. You can't throw out poisons and potential poisons, but you can "poison-proof" your home—that is, eliminate the dangers of accidental poisonings.

The fundamentals of poison-proofing are simple and sensible: recognize the dangerous substances in your home, handle them properly, and keep them in safe places. Although the fundamentals sound easy, some of the suggestions for poison-proofing your home may seem like inconveniences; you'll have to measure any inconvenience against the safety involved. The size of your home, the size of your family, and your family's day-to-day habits must all be taken into consideration. You'll have to decide which suggestions apply to your situation.

Control the number of dangerous substances

Even the smallest apartment can come to contain an astonishing number of medicines and household products. The narrow shelves of medicine cabinets can be made to house small drugstores; cupboards make room for every sort of cleaning product; closets hide items bought for some special need and then stored away because they might be needed again in the future.

Which products do you really need? The first step in poison-proofing your home can be a good spring cleaning. Throw away those products you no longer use or probably won't use in the near future. Most household products deteriorate with time, so holding onto them makes no sense. If you do need them again, you'll be better off buying new ones. You'll appreciate the empty spaces they leave behind, and your home will be safer.

Having cleaned out the old products, use care in buying new ones. Don't buy products that contain dangerous chemicals unless you truly need them, buy

Storing leftover chemicals

Many people are tempted to store leftover automobile, household, hobby, or garden chemicals in empty food containers. This is extremely dangerous even if the new contents are clearly marked on the container—children can't be expected to read labels, and adults will recognize the shape of the container and may overlook the label.

them in the smallest amounts possible, and—if you have a choice—buy the least toxic. And, of course, don't save any leftovers unless you plan to use the product again soon and can store it safely.

Store dangerous substances in assigned locations

You should know the exact location of every dangerous substance in your home. Every medicine and every household product should have a place and should be in its place when not in use. This will help you determine whether or not something is missing. As we'll see, all dangerous substances should be kept locked up.

Keep all dangerous substances in their original containers

Original containers are of crucial importance: they identify the product and contain valuable information on how the product should be used.
• Always keep medicine in the container it came in. That way, it won't be mistaken for something else, and you'll have the label and the directions.
• Never transfer a dangerous substance to a cup or beverage bottle or anything that might suggest that the contents are something to eat or drink. Children identify products by their containers—and so do adults.

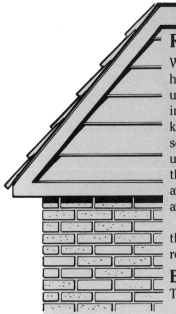

Room-by-room poison-proofing

Where you keep the dangerous substances in your home will be determined in large part by where you use them: for example, bathroom cleansers are stored in the bathroom, kitchen cleansers are stored in the kitchen. This is more than convenient—it makes good sense to keep dangerous products near where they're used. That way, you won't have to carry them around the house (and risk leaving them out if you're called away to do something else), and you can put them away easily after using them.

Room-by-room poison-proofing means recognizing the dangers presented by the substances used in each room and storing these substances safely.

Bathroom

The best place to begin poison-proofing your home

Is it clearly labeled?
Make sure everything in the medicine cabinet is clearly labeled. If a label is coming off, tape it back on or make another label; if a product has lost its label and you don't know what it is, throw it out.

• If a label becomes torn or soiled, repair or clean it. Secure loose labels with transparent adhesive tape, and repair or replace torn labels. If you absolutely must transfer a product to a different container, label the new container—and don't let any of the container's old label show.

Use childproof tops

Childproof tops are available for most medicines and many household products (see pages 13 to 15). Use them, and remember:
• Refasten the safety closure immediately after each use.
• Childproof tops may lose their effectiveness after repeated use, so don't try to reuse them—request new packaging when you get prescriptions refilled.

Be prepared

Know the number of your poison control center, and make sure it's located on or near every phone in your home. Keep a 1-oz bottle of ipecac syrup in the medicine cabinet.

Don't lock the medicine cabinet
Because the medicine cabinet contains emergency first-aid products—including ipecac syrup—you shouldn't lock it. Since you shouldn't lock it, you shouldn't use it to store anything dangerous if you have children under age 5.

Warning labels

The telephone stickers distributed by some poison control centers make handy warning labels for storage places used for dangerous substances. If you have children, you may decide to use the special warning labels such as "Mr. Yuk" (see pages 28 to 29).

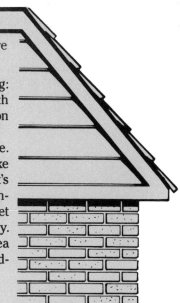

is the bathroom, site of that little storage place we call the medicine cabinet.

The medicine cabinet. The name is misleading: a medicine cabinet is a very poor place to keep both prescription medicines and many nonprescription medicines. There are two good reasons for this:
• Accessibility. Medicine cabinets are too accessible. They're usually located over the sink, and sinks make handy stepping-stones for exploring children. What's more, because every family member uses the bathroom daily, anything you put in your medicine cabinet becomes readily available to everyone in your family. Better to use your medicine cabinet as a storage area for such items as toothpaste, deodorants, and adhesive bandages, rather than medicines.

continued

Room-by-room poison-proofing
continued

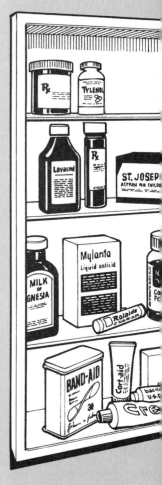

• Atmosphere. A bathroom's warm, moist atmosphere isn't good for some medicines: it can cause them to deteriorate. The labels of many medicines state that the medicine should be kept in a cool, dry place, and few bathrooms are cool and dry.

Use your medicine cabinet to store products used daily or necessary to deal with emergencies. Make use of the varying heights of the cabinet's shelves: the most commonly used (and least likely to cause harm) items on the lower shelves; those that are potentially dangerous on the higher shelves. Thus, your bottom shelves might contain first-aid items (such as sterile gauze, adhesive bandages, absorbent cotton, antiseptics, and antibacterial ointments); the middle shelves could contain nonprescription medications for the treatment of such symptoms as diarrhea or stomach upset; the top shelves could be used for such emergency products as ipecac syrup.

Don't let your medicine cabinet become a "mini" drugstore. Keep track of what's in it, and clean it out periodically—at least every 6 months.

Some drug products lose their potency with the passage of time, particularly after they've been opened; others change in consistency (for example, Milk of Magnesia dries out if it's been opened and left on the shelf too long). Many drugs have an expiration date printed on their labels. Get rid of all drugs that have become outdated or gone bad (liquids change color or consistency or become cloudy; tablets become crumbly).

Dispose of old drug products by pouring them down the drain or flushing them down the toilet (unless

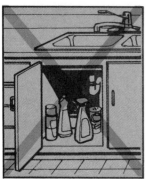

Kitchen
The first step in poison-proofing your kitchen is dividing its contents into foods and nonfoods.
• Store foods and nonfoods in separate cupboards. Label the outside of cupboards containing nonfoods with warning labels, and lock them if possible. If you must store foods and nonfoods together, keep them on different shelves.
• Keep all nonfood items out of the sight and reach of children. Where you keep these items will change as your children grow (see pages 31 to 32).

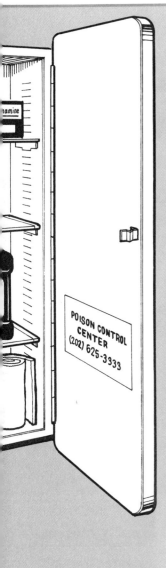

POISON CONTROL CENTER (202) 625-3333

the label instructions indicate other disposal methods). Rinse the container before discarding it.

Throw out the old containers—never reuse a medicine container for another product.

Both prescription and nonprescription drugs should be kept in a cool, dry place out of the sight and reach of children and away from food and other household products. Many people choose to keep their medicines on a high shelf in a hall or bedroom closet. This is acceptable if there are no children in your home, but if you have children—or if children frequently visit—you'll want to find a safer place.

• Locked cabinet or closet. The best place to store dangerous medicines is in a locked cabinet or closet. This cabinet or area of the closet should contain only medicines. Don't store medicines together with other household products, and don't store medicines together with food items.

• Locked box. Many people use locked boxes—a tackle box works well—instead of a cabinet or closet. You can keep prescription and nonprescription drugs in separate boxes. Label the outside of each box with a list of what's inside. This will make it easier to find specific medicines, which can be important in an emergency.

Cupboard. The medicine cabinet isn't the only storage place in most bathrooms. There may be a cupboard in your bathroom—perhaps it's beneath the sink. This is a handy place to store the products, such as tile cleaner and toilet bowl cleaner, you use in the bathroom, but it's not safe unless it's locked.

Never leave products on open shelves or on the rim of the bathtub.

• Use safety latches or locks on all cupboards and storage areas where nonfood items are stored. It's particularly important to keep the more dangerous substances—such as drain cleaners, tile cleaners, and products containing ammonia—locked up.

Don't use windowsills, counter tops, or the top of the refrigerator to "hide" medicines or potentially dangerous household products. Children are capable of reaching almost anything they can see. What's more, another adult—or a tall youth—may relocate the object in your absence.

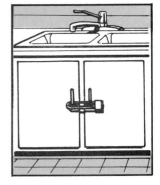

Room-by-room poison-proofing
continued

Throughout the house

Don't use poisonous plants as indoor decorations (see page 92), and try to keep all plants out of the reach of young children—even plants that aren't poisonous can make a child sick if he or she eats enough of them.

Make sure all alcoholic beverages are out of sight and out of reach of children, and keep ashtrays empty and out of reach.

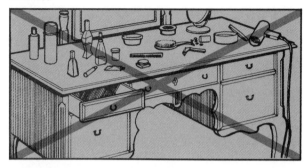

Similar containers

Always keep medicines apart from other household products because containers may look enough alike to cause confusion. Remember that the containers of prescription medicines may also look very much alike, particularly if you have all your prescriptions filled by the same pharmacy. Always read the label.

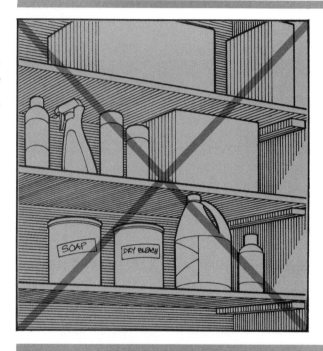

The garage floor

Antifreeze smells good and tastes sweet. It's also deadly if enough is ingested. Keep containers of antifreeze securely stored, and if you drain the antifreeze from your car, don't leave it lying on your garage floor or driveway. Both children and pets have been seriously poisoned from drinking antifreeze off the ground. If you drain your car's antifreeze, dispose of it properly—it should go directly into a sewer. Don't pour it into the ground (it might pollute the water supply), and don't let it stand in gutters. It evaporates very slowly and endangers children and animals.

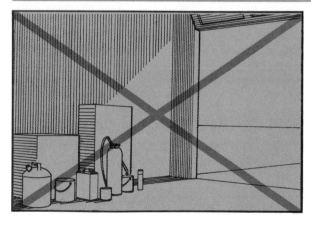

Bedroom

Clean all medicines and cosmetics off bedside tables or dressers. Lock up the medicines, and put the cosmetics where children can't see or reach them. Keeping such products within easy reach may seem handy, but it's very dangerous, both to children and to you.

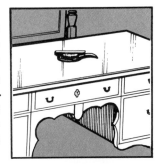

If you keep medicines in a dresser drawer, make sure it's locked. Children like to examine their parents' belongings; a child trying on his father's ties shouldn't be allowed to try his father's medicine.

Laundry, workshop, basement

Bleaches, soaps, detergents, fabric softeners, bluing agents, spray starches—all laundry products—should be kept out of sight and reach of children, preferably in a locked cabinet.

Don't transfer these products to other containers.

Workshops and basements are frequently taken over by hobbyists, and many hobbies involve the use of dangerous chemicals. If you develop your own photographs, you've got dangerous chemicals; if you enjoy woodworking, you've probably got paints, glues, and varnishes around, all of which are dangerous.

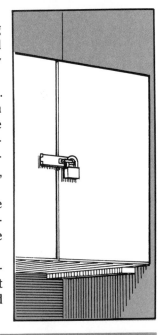

Many hobbyists develop bad habits—they store their chemicals in empty cups, use unlabeled containers, and leave these various supplies out where anyone can get at them.

The best solution, of course, is to keep the chemicals locked up. If that proves impossible, try to put a lock on the hobby-room door and keep it locked when the hobbyist's away.

Garage

The garage is the only proper place for a host of chemicals, such as paints and varnishes, turpentine, kerosene, gasoline, antifreeze, insecticides, and herbicides. In addition, you may have flower bulbs (some can be dangerous), other gardening supplies, or swimming pool chemicals in your garage.

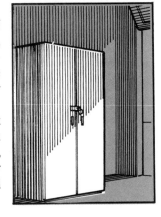

All of these chemicals and supplies must be kept in a locked cabinet, and they should all be kept in their original containers. If you have an outdoor shed, use it to house those items that aren't bothered by subfreezing temperatures. Keep its door locked, and put a warning label on it.

Tips for handling medicines properly

Follow these precautions when handling prescription and nonprescription medicines, including vitamins and minerals:

• Keep all medicines out of the sight and reach of children, preferably locked up.

• Keep all medicines in child-resistant safety containers (always ask for safety tops on prescription medicines and look for those nonprescription medicines that come in childproof containers).

• Never use medicine from an unlabeled bottle. If a medicine has lost its label, throw it out.

• Secure loose labels with transparent adhesive tape, and repair or replace torn labels.

• Give medicine only to the person designated on the prescription label.

• If your child takes a specific medicine, check with your doctor before giving him or her another medicine, even a nonprescription product like aspirin.

• Never give or take medicine in the dark.

• Always pay attention to what you're doing when measuring medicine.

• Call all medicines by their proper names, and never refer to them as candy.

• Don't make a game of giving medicine.

• Don't take medicine in front of a child—he or she may try to imitate you.

• Flush unused or outdated medicine down the toilet or pour it down the sink (unless the container gives other disposal directions). Rinse out the container and discard it where it's out of the reach of children and pets.

• Never take more than the prescribed or indicated dosage of any medicine. More won't make you feel better faster, and it may injure you.

• Avoid accidental overdoses—keep a record of medicines given to children or allow only one person to administer medicine. Many children have received overdoses because both parents gave them the same medication and neither was aware of the other's action.

• Store all medicines separately from other household products.

• Keep all medicines in their original containers.

• Don't mix medicines; don't store different kinds of pills in the same container (this can lead to confusion, and some medicines are capable of absorbing the potency of others).

• Don't save prescription medicines. Get rid of them as soon as the illness for which they were prescribed is over or the prescribing regimen is completed. Getting rid of them removes a possible hazard; furthermore, over a period of time, chemical changes can take place in the medicine that render it useless or even dangerous.

• Never use an old medicine to treat apparently similar symptoms occurring months or years later.

• Never take a medicine prescribed for a friend or relative who had the same complaint.

• Don't give medicines prescribed for one child to another child.

• Make sure the name of the drug appears on all prescription labels for rapid identification.

• Don't store containers of similar size, shape, and labeling near one another.

• Never allow anyone else, even an older child, to get medicine for you.

• Don't drink medicines from the bottle. This is a poor way to measure dosages, and if a child sees you, he or she might try to imitate you.

More tips for poison-proofing your home

The importance of labels

Product and medicine labels contain valuable information: what the product or medicine is; what it's made of; how it should be used, including safety precautions; and how much of the product or medicine is in the container. Many labels also include expiration dates, and there may be special information for the proper disposal of the product or medicine.

Always read the label before using any medicine or household product. No matter how many times you've taken the medicine or used the product, read the label before each use. Many medicine containers and household products look alike—if you don't check the label, you may take the wrong medicine or use a product improperly.

Labels are of great importance for another reason: they provide information that can be essential in the event of a poisoning accident. If you have the label, you'll know what substance was taken, and you may also be able to determine how much was taken.

Caution: Many labels include suggested antidotes—such information may be inaccurate or out of date. In the event of a poisoning emergency, follow the instructions of your poison control center, doctor, or hospital emergency room.

What is it?

No home is big enough to have room for unidentifiable products. If you don't know what something is (because it has lost its label or its label has become illegible), throw it out.

Industrial strength

Think twice before buying "industrial-strength" products. If the chemicals in the product really are strong enough to be used in industry, they don't belong in your home.

Is it still safe to use?

If a product doesn't have an expiration date, put a label on the container with the date of purchase and the date it was first opened. If there are any questions in the future, a pharmacist can tell you whether or not the product is safe to use. This applies to all drug products, but pay special attention to iodine, eye drops, eye washes, nose drops, cough remedies, and ointments—in addition to losing potency, such products can become harmful with age.

Cabinets, cupboards, closets

Keeping things locked up in cabinets, cupboards, or closets may make it hard for you to find what you want. There's a simple solution to this problem: attach a list of what you've put inside to the outside of each storage area. Don't forget to put a warning sticker on the outside of areas used to store dangerous substances.

Keeping foods away from nonfoods

A food is anything suitable to eat; a nonfood is anything not suitable to eat. By definition, the two are very different—in reality, however, they're sometimes very similar. Many nonfood products look like foods: bleach, for example, looks like soda. If you put bleach in an empty soft-drink bottle, you'll be endangering everyone around you—and not just the children. This is one important reason for keeping all products—food and nonfood—in their original containers.

Even containers, however, can cause confusion. Many food containers resemble nonfood containers, so storing food containers near nonfood containers is dangerous. Keep in mind the simple fact that young children can't read and are intrigued by attractive containers. A child in search of cookies will investigate any available container—and may sample the contents. Even an adult—particularly one in a hurry or thinking about other things—can mistake a nonfood container for a food container.

Family size

Unless you have a very large family or you're buying a product you use frequently, there's no sense in buying "family size" containers. It may seem like a bargain when you buy it, but it'll seem like a waste when you have to throw away the unused, spoiled remains.

4

Children and Poisons

When children come in contact with poisons, the result can be tragic. Such tragedies are all the more heartbreaking because they're preventable. The way to prevent accidental poisonings is to keep children and poisons apart.

Children as victims

Why do so many accidental poisonings happen to children under age 5? Children under age 5 are by nature potential poisoning victims—they'll put everything and anything into their mouths.

Children under age 5 are full of boundless curiosity. Newly arrived in our world, they're tireless and fearless explorers, and one of the ways they learn about our world is by taste. Anything within a child's reach may end up in that child's mouth.

Children are also great imitators: they like to do what they see other people, particularly their parents, do. If they see a parent take medicine, they'll be eager to do the same.

Until they're taught otherwise, children don't know that certain substances can hurt them. They have no notion of danger. And, of course, they can't read. To a child under age 5, a package of rat poison looks very much like a package of cookies.

Children need to be protected, and only adults can do that job.

Poison-proofing, childproofing

You can't watch over your children every moment of every day, but you can make your home safe, and you can teach your children the attitudes and behaviors that will help them avoid accidents.

Making your home safe means poison-proofing it. Follow the guidelines given on pages 18 to 23 for poison-proofing your home. The fundamentals of poison-proofing include:

• limiting the number of dangerous substances in your home

• storing all dangerous substances in assigned locations, and keeping all dangerous substances locked up

• keeping all dangerous substances in their original containers.

How many poisonings occur?
Determining the number of poisonings that occur each year is very difficult. The most reliable figures are those gathered from poison control centers, but such figures don't reflect the true number of poisonings. Many poisonings are treated by private doctors or by hospitals without poison control centers, and such poisonings frequently go unreported.

What do poisons taste like?
Taste isn't important: children will drink or eat large quantities of the worst-tasting substances. For example, a child will chew and swallow—without the aid of water—aspirin tablets.

These measures become even more important if you have children. In fact, if you have children or if children frequently visit your home, you'll want to combine these measures with further "child-proofing" measures. The basic philosophy of child-proofing is "out of sight, out of reach, and locked up."

"Keep out of the reach of children"

You've probably seen the phrase hundreds of times: "Keep out of the reach of children." The question is, how far can a child reach?

Children can reach as far as if not farther than adults. They reach "farther" by getting into places no adult would dream of going. A cupboard full of common household products isn't exciting to an adult, but to a child it's a wonderland to be explored. Putting something in the back of a closet isn't putting it out of children's reach.

Putting dangerous substances on high shelves isn't enough either: if a child can see something, he or she may try to reach it. And regardless of their relatively small sizes, children can usually find a way to reach whatever they can see.

Never underestimate your child's cleverness and skill in getting to poisons. Doctors treating cases of accidental poisonings of children frequently hear such phrases from parents as "I had no idea he could get to it." They never thought their child could perform such skills as opening doors, unscrewing caps, climbing shelves, prying off tops, opening purses, and remembering where poisons were kept.

Never underestimate your child's speed. Children can move with amazing speed: they can grab a package and open it very quickly.   .

Thus, "keep out of the reach of children" means several things:
• Keep all dangerous substances locked up.
• When you're using dangerous substances around a small child, never let the substance out of your sight. If you have to answer the phone or the doorbell, take the substance with you. Put dangerous substances back as soon as you've finished using them. And be alert when putting away groceries or cooking dinner—anytime you're distracted and you've got potentially dangerous substances out.

Safety catches

If you have a child, you've probably already "child-proofed" your home—put special covers over electric

Dangers in purses
Keep your purse out of your child's reach, and be sure to tell all guests about this precaution. Keep in mind that your child may associate a purse with gum and candy. Many people keep medicine, perfume, and chemical sprays in their purses.

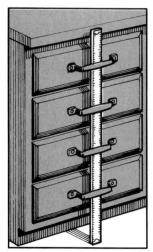

Be practical
Use your imagination to promote safety. Here, a yardstick secures kitchen drawers from an inquisitive child.

Don't break your own rules
Your behavior is probably just as important as the rules you try to set. If your child sees you take vitamins every morning, he or she will come to believe that taking pills is correct; your rules about not touching any pills will have less force. Don't take any medicine—even vitamins—in front of children.

sockets, placed safety gates at the top of staircases, put covers over the sharp edges of furniture.

Several childproofing kits are available (one of the best-known brand names is KinderGard), and most include safety catches for cupboards, drawers, and doors. These are easy to open for adults but almost impossible for young children.

Safety catches are an essential part of child-proofing your home. They allow you to quickly and easily take out and put back dangerous household chemicals.

Educating children

The way you treat medicines and other potentially dangerous substances will influence the way your children treat them. Children are great imitators; they'll follow your example.

Giving medicine should never be made into a game. Don't call medicines candy, and don't tell a child a medicine tastes delicious. When giving flavored or brightly colored medicine to children, always refer to it as medicine. Children should regard medicines seriously, but matter-of-factly.

You can protect children in your home, but you can't go with them everywhere. Be careful, then, to help them develop a sensible attitude toward potentially dangerous substances. You should teach children not to eat or drink anything that hasn't been given to them by parents or others in authority. In particular, they should be taught not to eat berries, flowers, seeds, or leaves—any plant part—they find inside or outside the home.

And don't break your own rules—adults suffer accidental poisonings, too.

Wordless warning labels

Wordless warning labels were created in an effort to prevent accidental poisonings among children. They're symbols designed to turn children away from potential poisons.

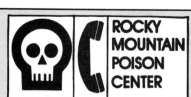

ROCKY MOUNTAIN POISON CENTER

303/629-1123 1-800/332-3073
DENVER METRO   OUTSIDE METRO DENVER

Emergency label
The copyrighted logo of the American Association of Poison Control Centers is for use by its members as a means of identifying itself and member poison control centers.

Iron supplements

Dietary supplements containing iron (ferrous sulfate, ferrous gluconate, ferrous fumarate) are among the most frequently overlooked potential poisons. An acute overdose of iron can cause corrosive damage to the stomach and small intestine, blood circulation problems, damage to the liver and other organs, shock, and even death.

Young children have been seriously injured by swallowing doses of 200 to 400 mg of iron. This is equivalent to 14 to 27 children's vitamin-and-mineral supplements with iron (15 mg each) or 4 to 7 tablets of a typical adult iron supplement (60 mg each, a common dosage for pregnant women).

Iron supplements are found in every drugstore and can be bought without a prescription. Unfortunately, the tablets are usually brightly colored and look like candy to young children. Never leave any vitamins, minerals, or iron supplements within reach of children—treat these pills like medicines.

Mouthwashes

Mouthwashes, common in many homes, are responsible for frequent poisonings of children under age 5. These products contain alcohol, come in containers without child-resistant tops, are often brightly colored and sweet tasting, and are frequently left within easy reach.

Selecting a symbol to use on a warning label for children isn't easy. The traditional skull and crossbones doesn't frighten all children: many associate it with pirates, horror movies, and exciting stories. Even the notion of "poison" doesn't necessarily frighten children, who, after all, have only the vaguest understanding of death.

Some poison control centers have designed wordless warning labels and made them available to the public. But your child won't be safe if you just slap these stickers on all the potential poisons in your home: you must involve your child in the operation, instructing him or her in the meaning of the symbol. This procedure is to teach the child not to put anything into his or her mouth without approval from an adult.

Wordless warning labels have drawbacks. Some children are attracted to them. Furthermore, taking a child around the house and pointing out dangerous substances may only increase his or her curiosity. Finally, children who've been taught to look for a warning label are in danger when they visit friends or relatives who don't use the labels; a child who has learned to look for a certain label may believe a product is safe because it has no label.

Some children respond well to wordless warning labels—they understand that the symbol means "don't touch." Many parents have reported that such labels have prevented possible poisonings.

Whether or not you use warning labels is up to you. Even if you decide not to use the warning labels designed for children, such as "Mr. Yuk" or "Officer Ugg," you should make use of the telephone stickers distributed by some poison control centers. You can use these to label the outside of cabinets or boxes containing medicines or household products. Use one on or near every telephone in your home. It's also a good idea to put the poison control center's number on the inside of your medicine cabinet.

When do poisonings occur?

An accidental poisoning can occur at any time, and poison control centers report that the volume of calls they receive remains about the same throughout the day. However, the centers' records show that the number of calls increases slightly between the hours of 4 p.m. and 8 p.m.; in particular, the number of calls rises between the hours of 4 p.m. and 6 p.m. This last period has become infamous as the "arsenic hour." It's when parents come home from work and prepare dinner and children are hungry and cranky.

You should always be alert to your child's activities, but you should be particularly alert when your family's normal routine is disrupted or when you're distracted. Examples of such periods are:

- when you have an illness in the family
- when you're cooking a meal
- when your family is moving
- when you have family tension
- when a guest is in your home or you're giving a party (remember to caution guests about where they put their purses)
- when your child is hungry or tired
- when you're on a trip
- during holidays.

How many poisoning opportunities do you see?

The greatest number of poisonings occur between 4 p.m. and 6 p.m., when children are tired, bored, hungry, and indoors, and adults are preoccupied. In this scene, the children can easily reach three possible poisonous substances—vitamins with iron, a poisonous plant, and cleaning supplies under the sink.

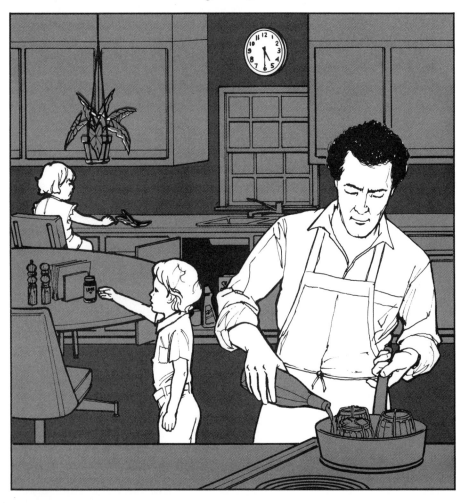

As your child grows

Each stage of a child's growth brings new joys to parents—and presents new dangers of poisoning accidents. Remember that each new skill your child develops calls for greater vigilance on your part.

Birth to 7 months

During their first 7 months, babies learn to roll over and reach for objects; by age 7 months, most have learned to sit up and crawl. Babies will put almost anything into their mouths.

* Make certain the ingredients used in your baby's formula are kept in clearly labeled containers to avoid the possibility of mixing a harmful substance into the formula, such as salt instead of sugar.
* Don't overmedicate your baby. When giving medicine, always follow the directions on the label or your doctor's instructions. Avoid accidental overdoses: many children are given too much medicine because both parents gave the same medication to the child and neither was aware of the other's action.
* Keep all medicines and household products away from your baby. Return medicines and household products to safe places immediately after use. Never set down anything near your baby "for just a moment"—babies learn to grab things and can move with unexpected speed.
* Never permit another child to give medicine to your baby.
* Begin now to put all potentially dangerous substances in locked cabinets or boxes, or at the very least on high shelves. Don't store dangerous household products under the sink or on low shelves.
* Carefully sterilize your baby's formula and promptly refrigerate milk and opened jars of baby food to prevent the growth of harmful bacteria in these foods.
* Don't let your baby eat or chew on plants or parts of plants.

7 to 12 months

Babies at this age learn to crawl, pull themselves up to stand, and may even learn to walk holding onto a support. They put everything within reach into their mouths and pull things down.

* Always return medicines and household products to a locked cabinet or high shelf immediately after use.
* If you must store household products in a low cupboard (such as that beneath the sink), lock the cup-

Is it sugar or salt?
Some nonpoisonous food substances can be harmful when given to an infant by mistake: for example, putting salt instead of sugar into a baby's formula. If you transfer items such as sugar and salt to another container, be sure to label the new container, and read the label before using the container's contents.

Children's medicines
Medicines prescribed for children aren't less dangerous than medicines prescribed for adults. Children's chewable vitamins with iron and baby aspirin are dangerous. Many of these are made to please children: they have sweet tastes and pretty colors. They are medicines: never give your child more than the prescribed or indicated dosage, make sure your child knows it's medicine, and keep these products locked up.

The terrible twos
When asked to name the
worst stage their children
went through, most parents
vote for the "terrible
twos"—terrible because
these children get into medicine cabinets and onto the
tops of dressers. These
children are most likely to
get into such things as
cleaning and polishing
products, petroleum prod-
ucts, turpentine, and paint.
That's because such materials are frequently stored
under bathroom or kitchen
sinks or in other cupboards
just at the eye level of a
toddler. Keep such areas
locked.

The age of accidents
Doctors refer to the period
between ages 1 and 3 as
the "age of accidents."

board or use safety closures (such as KinderGard locks).

1 to 3 years

Toddlers—children between the ages of 1 and 3—have the highest accident rate of any age group. They're zealous explorers: they climb, open doors and drawers, and reach for everything in sight. And they put everything they reach into their mouths. They have no sense of danger and need to be very carefully supervised. However, they're beginning to have a better understanding of what adults say to them, so this is a good time to begin teaching and enforcing safety rules. Remember that children at this age avidly imitate parents and other adults.

• Continue the same precautions as before and be especially alert: your child will eat anything—and climb to great heights to get it.

• Don't leave glasses or bottles of alcoholic beverages where your child can get at them.

• Don't take medicines in front of your child.

• Never get your child to take medicine by saying that it's candy or tastes delicious. Your child understands what you're saying and may search for the tasty "candy" when you're not looking.

• You may decide now to begin using wordless warning labels, such as "Mr. Yuk."

3 to 5 years

This is the age of the climber, so high cabinets or shelves are no longer safe; all medicines and dangerous products must be kept locked up.

• Follow the previous precautions.

• If you haven't already done so, you may decide to begin using wordless warning labels, such as "Mr. Yuk." Pay attention to how your child responds: some children are attracted to these labels rather than turned away by them.

• You should be educating your child about the dangers of poisons; firmly teach your child that he or she should never eat anything without an adult's approval. This includes all berries, seeds, nuts, or plant parts. It also includes paint chips.

Lead poisoning

Lead is contained in a variety of products, but it's usually associated with paint. Until about 40 years ago, all house paint was manufactured with some amount of lead.

Lead facts

• *Lead was added to paint for several reasons. The addition of lead made the paint dry faster and gave it a shinier and harder finish. In fact, the more lead, the better and more expensive the paint. Some paints contained as much as 50% lead.*

• *The "lead" in lead pencils is actually graphite, which is nontoxic.*

• *The first step in treating lead poisoning is to get the child away from the source of contamination. Locating the source of the lead isn't always easy: it may be in the child's home or a home or building the child visits frequently.*

• *Among the other potential sources of lead poisoning are water coming through lead pipes, juice kept in an improperly fired ceramic pitcher coated with lead-based glaze, painted furniture, color-tinted newspapers, and some painted toys.*

Medical scientists had known for many years that lead could be poisonous, and they eventually began to speak out against the presence of so much lead in our homes. Their efforts lead to the passage during the late 1970s of several laws regulating the amount of lead in paint.

These laws controlled the amount of lead in new paints but did nothing about the layers of dangerous lead-based paint remaining on the walls of millions of homes all across our country. This lead-based paint is responsible for most cases of lead poisoning: children eat it.

Why would children eat paint? Children suck and chew on toys and furniture (some of which may be covered with lead-based paint), and they'll pick at peeling paint and eat the chips they pull off. They may also come upon pieces of paint that fall to the floor; children will even gnaw the paint off windowsills.

Some children develop what is known as pica, an appetite for things other than food. A child with this tendency will actually crave paint chips—which unfortunately have a sweetish taste. Finally, lead-based paint is frequently present in older buildings, particularly those in inner-city areas inhabited by the disadvantaged. Many victims of lead poisoning are children whose parents can't afford to feed them—the children eat the paint because they're hungry.

Symptoms of lead poisoning

The symptoms of lead poisoning are subtle and may be confused with other things. Common symptoms include:

• listlessness (occurs early)
• irritability (occurs early)
• clumsiness
• loss of appetite and weight (occurs early)
• constipation (occurs early)
• a bluish line in the gums (occurs early)
• vomiting
• stomach cramps.

More lead facts
• *The paint in your home can be tested for lead. The usual method requires use of a meter that's placed against the wall to measure the amount of lead in the paint. This test can be performed by local health authorities: contact the nearest office of the U.S. Department of Health, Education, and Welfare.*

• *A chip of lead-based paint about the size of a fingernail contains almost 100 times the amount of lead that can safely be consumed in 1 day. If a child eats an average of three fingernail-sized chips a day for several months, he or she will become sick. The more lead the child eats, the more serious the effect.*

• *If you can't afford to repaint, keep your floors swept and look around to find paint that might be pulled off—brush off the loose paint with a broom or strong brush. If you can, scrape down the walls to get off all the old paint.*

• *A child with pica will eat such things as paint chips, plaster, crayons, chalk, wallpaper, newspaper (especially tinted), dirt, and cigarettes. Pica isn't restricted to children: pregnant women frequently develop pica.*

What happens in lead poisoning

Lead poisoning is a chronic poisoning. When a child ingests lead, his or her body absorbs about 10% to 15% of the metal and slowly excretes the rest. Most of the absorbed lead is retained in the child's bones; smaller quantities are stored in bone marrow, soft tissues, and red blood cells. If the child continues to ingest lead, large amounts will accumulate and eventually reach a toxic level.

Children may ingest lead for 3 to 6 months before anyone notices symptoms of lead poisoning. If a case of lead poisoning isn't identified and treated, and the source eliminated, the toxic lead levels in the child's body may cause serious complications, such as mental retardation. Lead poisoning can be fatal.

Treatment of lead poisoning

If you suspect that a child is suffering lead poisoning, take him or her to a doctor immediately. A simple blood test will determine whether or not the child's blood has too much lead.

A child with enough absorbed lead in his or her body to show symptoms will probably require hospitalization. Treatment usually consists of the administration of medicines to help the body rid itself of the lead.

Prevention of lead poisoning

Keep cribs away from windows that may be painted with lead-based paint, and be alert for any signs that your child is picking at painted surfaces. When you teach your children not to eat anything they find, indoors or outdoors, be clear that you mean everything, even things as small as paint chips.

Keep an eye on children outdoors—many exterior house paints, especially around windows, flake off easily.

Use only lead-free paint when you paint your home or anything in your home. And watch out for peeling paint: if your home is old enough, it may have layers of old, lead-based paint beneath the more recent layers of paint. If you suspect the presence of lead-based paint, scrape off all the layers of old or peeling paint before repainting with lead-free paint. Don't just add another coat of paint.

If your child has cravings for nonfood substances, he or she may have pica and must be well protected: persistent pica can cause lead or other poisoning. Discuss the problem with your doctor.

5 The Poisoning Emergency

The poisoning emergency
Here's what to do when you know or suspect that a poisoning has occurred.

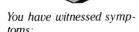

You have witnessed symptoms:
• *When did the symptoms begin?*
• *What are they?*

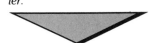

Find evidence, such as an open bottle or parts of a plant, or see the poisoning occur.

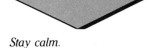

Stay calm.

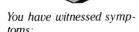

Call the poison control center.

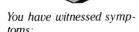

Follow instructions.

Whom to call
If you don't have access to your emergency numbers, dial 911 or the operator, explain what has happened, and ask for the number of the nearest hospital emergency room.

Despite your poison-prevention efforts, an accidental poisoning may occur. You can't foresee how or when such an accident might occur, but you can be prepared to handle poisoning accidents. Although they are medical emergencies and require immediate care, most accidental poisonings can be treated at home—with advice from a poison control center, doctor, or hospital emergency room—without a visit to a hospital.

How to recognize a poisoning
The first step in treating an accidental poisoning is recognizing that a poisoning has occurred. In many cases, this is quite simple—you'll see a child grab a container and eat or drink its contents. Or, if you don't actually see the poisoning accident take place, you may find telltale evidence that a poisoning has occurred:
• an open medicine or household chemical container
• spilled liquid, powder, or pills
• liquid, powder, or pills in the victim's mouth or on his teeth
• stains on the victim's clothing
• a peculiar odor on the victim's breath, body, or clothes
• burns or swelling on the victim's hands or mouth
• symptoms that might indicate a poisoning (see below).

You may become aware of an accidental poisoning in other ways: your child may tell you what he or she has done, or someone else may report it to you.

Never wait for symptoms to develop. If you have reason to suspect that a poisoning has occurred, call your poison control center immediately.

Symptoms of a poisoning
You may not see the poisoning take place, and you may have no reason to suspect that a poisoning has occurred. Instead, the victim may suddenly begin to show symptoms of a poison. (The sudden appearance of symptoms is an indication in itself of a poisoning.) Such symptoms include:

Remember the speed limit

If you're told to take the victim to a hospital emergency room, stay calm. Speed is essential, but don't overdo it. If you take off on a mad dash through traffic, you'll endanger yourself, the victim, and everyone in your path.

Nontoxic substances

If the substance involved is one of those listed as nontoxic (see page 91), you probably have nothing to worry about. But don't take chances: call the poison control center to make sure.

Have the following information ready when you call the poison control center, doctor, or emergency room:

1. the age and weight of the victim
2. the name of the product involved and its ingredients (or, if it's a plant, the kind of plant)
3. the amount of the poison or plant the victim has ingested
4. the time the poisoning occurred
5. any symptoms the victim may have, such as whether or not he has vomited.

You may be asked for further information, such as whether or not the victim suffers from any medical problems (diabetes, epilepsy, or high blood pressure, for example), and what medicines, if any, he takes regularly.

Follow the instructions of the poison control center, doctor, or emergency room. Remember: first-aid procedures differ according to the kind of poison involved, how the poison entered the body, the victim's weight, how long the poison has been in the victim, and other factors. Only expert medical personnel can determine the correct procedure. If you attempt to treat the victim yourself without expert advice, you may do further harm.

You may be told to take the victim to a hospital emergency room immediately. Take with you the following:

• The poison container and any of its remaining contents, or parts of the plant if a plant was involved. Such materials will help doctors identify the poison and estimate how much of it the victim swallowed.

• If a plant was involved, take enough of it for identification—for example, an entire mushroom or a branch with leaves, flowers, and berries.

• If the victim has vomited, take a container of the vomit. The vomit can be tested to determine the nature of the poison and, if undigested pills are vomited, the doctor may be able to determine how many the victim took.

• If possible, have another person drive while you keep the victim comfortable. Have a vomiting victim lie on his side to keep his airway clear.

If you have the container the poison came in (or the plant, if a plant was involved), you have an enormous advantage in treating the poisoning. The poison control center will be able to recommend the appropriate first-aid procedures. Don't begin any first-aid procedures for an ingested poison until you have received specific instructions.

Identify the poison
Identification of the poison is very important in the successful treatment of a poisoning. If the poison involved can't be identified, medical personnel will rely on supportive treatment— they'll treat the symptoms.

Scars
For children, the emotional scars from an accident may last much longer than any physical scars.

Examine the victim
Examine the victim closely—you may find the residue of powder or liquid around the mouth or on the teeth.

- nausea or vomiting
- altered or difficult breathing
- diarrhea (perhaps with stomach cramps)
- changes in the size of the pupils (enlarged [dilated] or very small [constricted])
- changes in facial expression (dull, masklike appearance; facial twitching)
- drooling or excessive salivation
- excessive sweating
- altered state of awareness, delirium, or mental disturbances
- changes in skin color, particularly around the lips or fingernails
- burning sensations in the mouth, throat, or stomach
- altered heartbeat
- changes in body temperature
- coughing
- gassiness
- headache
- muscle spasms, convulsions, or general or partial paralysis
- difficulty hearing (the victim may have trouble hearing or may hear a constant buzzing or roaring)

Breath odors and poisons
In many cases, an ingested poison will have an effect on the victim's breath. Smell the breath of any poisoning victim (or suspected poisoning victim) and report any peculiar breath odors to the poison control center, doctor, or emergency room. The following list matches breath odors to possible poisons:

Odor	Poison
Sweet	Acetone
Bitter almonds	Cyanide
Stale tobacco	Nicotine
Pear-like	Chloral hydrate
Alcoholic	Alcohols
Gasoline-like	Petroleum-like products
Garliclike	Phosphorus, arsenic
Shoe polish-like	Nitrobenzene
Violets	Turpentine

38

Toxidromes

Doctors consider the possibility of poisoning whenever a child under age 5 displays unexplained symptoms. Doctors can sometimes determine the kind of poison involved based on the symptoms because many poisons cause specific symptoms. Such a group of symptoms is called a toxidrome (or toxicologic symptom complex); if the doctor can pinpoint the toxidrome, he or she may be able to determine the poison involved.

Repeat poisoning

The experience of being poisoned doesn't end a child's curiosity. According to statistics, children who've been poisoned once are more likely than other children to be poisoned again within 1 year. Be alert for this so-called repeat poisoning. Review your poison-prevention efforts, and teach your child about the dangers of poisons.

- loss of muscle control, clumsiness
- burned or damaged skin
- unusual breath odors
- color changes in urine or stool
- weakness or tiredness
- visual disturbances.

These and many other symptoms could indicate a poisoning—or any number of illnesses. Call your doctor. Try to recall precisely when the symptoms began, and make a thorough search of your home to uncover evidence that a poisoning has occurred.

Avoid panic

Most cases of accidental poisonings involve nontoxic substances or substances taken in small amounts that are harmless. Most can be treated at home and require no first-aid treatment at all, not even ipecac syrup.

But even if the poisoning is life-threatening, you can handle the situation properly if you keep yourself under control. This is particularly important if the victim (or suspected victim) is a child. Children take their cues from the adults around them. If you become excited, a child will do the same. You may then mistake the child's sudden excitement for unusual behavior—a symptom of poisoning.

A calm atmosphere will be very important if you're instructed to make the victim vomit, an unpleasant procedure, particularly for the victim. Explain what you're doing; use simple language and speak in a calm voice. If the victim is a child, select simple words, and whatever you do or say, do or say it calmly. Encourage conversation to draw the child's attention away from the frightening aspects of the situation.

6

First Aid for Poisonings

You may not have to do anything
Most accidental poisonings require no treatment at all or only water or milk; ipecac syrup is called for in fewer than 20% of accidental poisonings.

Your poison-prevention efforts should include preparation for the first-aid treatment of accidental poisonings. If you're prepared, you'll be able to handle any poisoning accidents in a calm, level-headed manner.

Follow these three important measures to be prepared for an accidental poisoning:
• Keep the phone number of your nearest poison control center handy.
• Keep a bottle of ipecac syrup.
• Be familiar with the first-aid procedures for accidental poisonings.

Poison control centers

Put the telephone number of your nearest poison control center on or near every telephone in your home. The stickers provided by some poison control centers make this easy.

Your treatment of most accidental poisonings and suspected poisonings begins with a telephone call to a poison control center, doctor, or hospital emergency room.

In the case of ingested poisons, you shouldn't attempt any first-aid measures until you've contacted a poison control center, doctor, or emergency room and received specific instructions.

In the case of inhaled poisons or poisons spilled on the skin or into the eyes, call only after carrying out the recommended first-aid procedures. With such poisonings, you must begin first-aid measures immediately. Minutes count, so you need to be familiar with the first-aid procedures before an accident occurs.

Learn the route to the hospital
What's the shortest route to the nearest 24-hour hospital emergency room? Learn it now if you're uncertain. If you have a car, drive there from your home when you have a chance, and do it again every year or so, just in case a street has been changed to one way or the entrance to the emergency room has been moved to another area of the hospital.

In the case of certain ingested poisons, the poison control center, doctor, or emergency room may instruct you to make the victim vomit with ipecac syrup. Don't give ipecac syrup unless you're instructed to do so.

In some cases, you may be instructed to take the victim to the nearest hospital emergency room. Remember to take with you the container the poison came in if you have it, a sample of the plant if a plant was involved, and any vomit from the victim.

Ipecac

Ipecac syrup is a thick, amber-colored liquid with an unpleasant smell. It will stay fresh for several years if you keep it tightly closed and stored at room temperature. Check the expiration date each time you check the products in your medicine cabinet (which should be at least every 6 months).

Anorexics and bulimics

Although harmless when taken in the dosages necessary to cause vomiting, ipecac syrup can be potentially deadly if used in very large amounts. In fact, in large enough amounts, one ingredient in ipecac (emetine) can cause irreversible damage to the heart. This damage can eventually lead to what appears to be a heart attack.

Many people suffering from anorexia nervosa and bulimia purposely misuse ipecac syrup. Anorexia is self-starvation; bulimia is recurrent binge eating followed by self-induced vomiting or purging by laxatives and diuretics. Both disorders are most frequently encountered in women in their early teens to 30s who attempt to drastically limit their intake of food in an obsessive desire to be extremely thin.

Pharmacists have been alerted to this problem, and ipecac syrup labels may soon include a warning about the dangers of using ipecac syrup incorrectly.

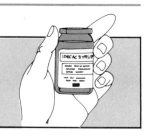

You can put the poison control center's telephone number on your bottle of ipecac syrup.

Ipecac syrup

Ipecac syrup is an emetic, a substance that makes people vomit. It comes from the dried roots of a shrub *(Cephaelis ipecacuanha)* native to South America.

The treatment for many swallowed poisons is to get the toxic substance out of the stomach before it's absorbed into the blood. To get the toxic substance out, you'll make the victim vomit, and ipecac syrup is a safe and sure way to make a victim vomit.

You should always keep on hand a 1-oz bottle of ipecac syrup. It's available without a prescription in most pharmacies for about $2.

Never give anyone ipecac syrup unless you're instructed to do so by a poison control center, doctor, or hospital emergency room. Not all poisoning emergencies require the removal of the poison from the stomach, and in some cases vomiting would be dangerous.

Ipecac syrup saves lives—according to some estimates, 150,000 every year. Yet ipecac syrup itself is a poison. That's why the instructions for its use allow only two doses; more may be toxic.

Using ipecac syrup

The dosages of ipecac syrup are different for infants and older people. The poison control center, doctor, or hospital emergency room will give you complete instructions. The following are the normal doses:
• If the victim is under age 1: 2 tsp followed by at least two to three glasses of water.
• If the victim is age 1 or older: 1 or 2 tbsp followed by at least two to three glasses of water.

Give water, not milk. Have the victim drink more water if possible. If the victim hasn't vomited within 20 minutes, you can repeat the dose of ipecac syrup. Do not give a third dose. If the victim doesn't vomit after the second dose, call the poison control center, doctor, or emergency room for further instructions.

Have the victim kneel, sit up, or lean forward while vomiting. If the victim is an infant, hold him or her in your lap. If possible, have the victim vomit into a

Effective vomiting
Vomiting is effective only if it's done within 4 hours of the ingestion of a solid substance or within 2 hours of the ingestion of a liquid.

When not to make the victim vomit
Poison victims shouldn't be made to vomit in certain cases because doing so could cause further damage or complications. Don't make the victim vomit in the following cases:
1. If the victim has swallowed an acid or alkali. Acids and alkalis burn the mouth and throat when they're swallowed, and they can produce more burning if they're vomited.
2. If the victim has swallowed a petroleum-like product. Petroleum-like products give off fumes that can cause a severe type of pneumonia if they're inhaled into the lungs during vomiting.
3. If the victim is unconscious or losing consciousness.
4. If the victim is having convulsions or has just had convulsions.
5. If the victim has pain or a burning sensation in the mouth or throat.
6. If the victim has a serious heart condition (the strain of vomiting could aggravate the condition).

large bowl or pot. You may need to take the vomit to the hospital for analysis.

You may be instructed to use other common household products (such as a mixture of flour and water) to treat accidental poisonings. Don't worry about what other products you should have on hand—if you have ipecac syrup, you'll be prepared to deal with most accidental poisonings.

In addition, learn the principles of first aid for accidental poisonings before a poisoning occurs. If you've reviewed the necessary steps in advance, you'll feel more sure of yourself and be calmer if you're ever called on to act.

General first aid for ingested (swallowed) poisons

1. Check for breathing and open the victim's airway. Loosen any tight clothing.
2. Start artificial respiration if the victim has stopped breathing.
3. Call for an ambulance, and call the poison control center, doctor, or hospital emergency room and follow all instructions.
4. Keep the victim warm.
5. If the victim is vomiting, turn his body and head to the side, and position him so the vomit runs out of his mouth instead of back into his stomach or into his lungs.
6. Save (and give to the doctor or emergency personnel) whatever caused the poisoning (remaining medicine, parts of plants, household products); you should also save any vomit.

First aid for ingested substances (neither corrosive nor petroleum-like)

1. Give 1 to 2 cups of water or milk if the victim is conscious and not having convulsions.
2. Call a poison control center, emergency room, or doctor for instructions.
3. If you're instructed to do so, give the victim ipecac syrup. Save any vomit for examination.
4. If the victim doesn't vomit after you've given ipecac syrup twice, call the poison control center, emergency room, or doctor for further advice.

Artificial respiration (mouth-to-mouth resuscitation)

1. Lay the victim on his back. Loosen tight clothing. Open the victim's airway by tilting his head back and chin up. To do this, use one hand to support his neck while you press backward on his forehead with your other hand. Look for the rise and fall of the chest, listen, and feel for breathing.

2. Keep the victim's head tilted back and pinch his nostrils shut with your thumb and forefinger. Take a deep breath and place your mouth firmly over the victim's open mouth. Breathe into his mouth four times, refilling your lungs after each breath. Give the breaths in rapid succession, and don't allow the victim's lungs to fully deflate.

2a. If the victim is under age 1, place your mouth over his nose and mouth, as shown.

3. Maintain the head tilt, and look, listen, and feel for air movement. If the victim still isn't breathing, form a tight seal and breathe in the cycle as follows:

• If the victim is an adult: breathe for the victim once every 5 seconds (12 times a minute).

• If the victim is an infant up to 1 year old: use gentle, small breaths once every 3 seconds (20 times a minute).

• If the victim is a child 1 year to 8 years old: breathe once every 4 seconds (15 times a minute).

Continue breathing for the victim until he is breathing on his own or help arrives. Many people have revived after hours of artificial respiration.

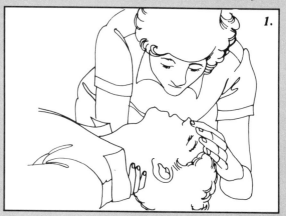

1.

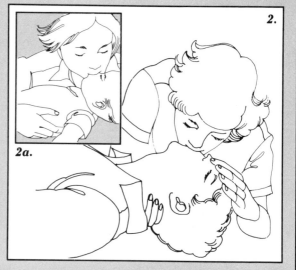

2.

2a.

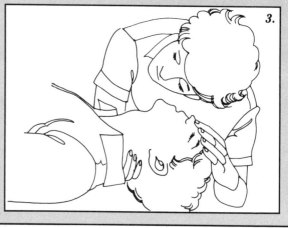

3.

⊞ First aid for ingested petroleum-like substances

If the victim has swallowed a petroleum-like product, immediately call a poison control center, emergency room, or doctor. Don't make the victim vomit unless you're told to do so.

These products often give a gasoline-like odor to the victim's breath.

⊞ First aid for ingested corrosive substances (acids and alkalies)

1. Immediately call a poison control center, doctor, or emergency room for first-aid instructions. Don't make the victim vomit.
2. Give 1 to 2 cups of water or milk if the victim is alert and can swallow.

Acids and alkalis often burn the face, mouth, and throat.

⊞ First aid for inhaled poisons

1. Move the victim away from the source of the poison to fresh air immediately.
2. Loosen the victim's clothing and open his airway.
3. If the victim isn't breathing, begin artificial respiration immediately. Don't stop until the victim is breathing well or help arrives.
4. Call a poison control center, doctor, or emergency room for further instructions.

Caution: If you're attempting to rescue someone from smoke, gas, or chemical fumes, follow these precautions:

1. If you're alone, call for help before you attempt to rescue the victim. You, too, may be overcome by smoke, gas, or fumes.
2. Don't light a match, turn on a light switch, or produce a flame or spark in the presence of gas or fumes.
3. Before entering the area, take several deep breaths of fresh air. Then inhale deeply and hold your breath as you go in.
4. Don't attempt any first-aid measures until you're in the fresh air.

⊞ First aid for poisons on the skin

Caution
Don't apply ointments unless you're instructed to do so by medical personnel.

Speed is essential: a delay of only seconds may greatly increase the injury. Remove the substance as quickly as possible: water dilutes it and flushes it away, and removal of contaminated clothing takes any absorbed chemicals away from the skin.

1. Remove any contaminated clothing, including shoes and socks. Also remove any jewelry, watches, or rings.
2. Flush the affected area immediately with large quantities of cool water from a shower, hose, faucet, or pail. Continue flushing for at least 15 minutes.
3. Cover the affected area with a loose, clean cloth.
4. Call a poison control center, doctor, or emergency room for further instructions. Call even if the affected area isn't large and isn't causing the victim any pain.

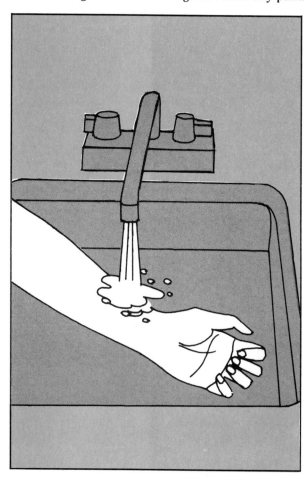

⊞ First aid for poisons in the eye

Don't take chances with eyes

Substances that wouldn't hurt the skin can damage an eye's delicate tissues. Don't take any risks. If you have any doubts about a substance, flush the eyes and get medical help.

Speed is essential: a delay of only seconds may greatly increase the injury.

1. Hold the victim's eyelids open with your fingers and rinse the eyes and face with a stream of water for at least 15 to 20 minutes.

● Use water from a faucet, drinking fountain, or hose, or use a glass or other container to pour water into the eye.

● Don't use an eye cup.

● Remove contact lenses or slide them gently onto the white of the eye, using the eyelids.

● Don't allow the victim to rub the eyes.

● Don't use eye drops, drugs, or ointments.

2. Call a poison control center, doctor, or emergency room for further advice—but don't delay the treatment.

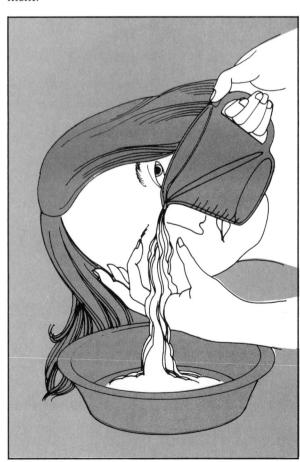

Protect uninjured eyes

If only one eye has been affected, turn the victim's head to one side, keeping the uninjured eye higher so that the chemical doesn't get into it.

Poison treatment chart

This chart presents the suggested treatments for several kinds of poisoning. The number after each substance refers to the appropriate treatment.

Caution: This chart can't replace your call to a poison control center, doctor, or hospital emergency room.

Suggested treatment:

1. Small amounts of this substance aren't poisonous, so no treatment is necessary.

2. Make the victim vomit. Give ipecac syrup in the following dosages:
If the victim is under 1 year of age:
Two teaspoons followed by at least 2 to 3 glasses of water.
If the victim is 1 year or older:
One or two tablespoons followed by at least 2 to 3 glasses of water.
Don't make the victim vomit if he or she is unconscious, or having convulsions. Call the poison control center, doctor, or emergency room for instructions.

3. Dilute or neutralize the poison with water or milk. Don't make the victim vomit. Call the poison control center, doctor, or emergency room.

4. Dilute or neutralize the poison with water or milk. Don't make the victim vomit. The substance may burn the mouth and throat. Call the poison control center, doctor, or emergency room.

5. Immediately rinse skin thoroughly with running water (see page 44). Continue for at least 15 minutes. Call the poison control center, doctor, or emergency room for help.

6. Immediately rinse eyes with running water (see page 45). Continue for 15 to 20 minutes. Call the poison control center, doctor, or emergency room for further instructions.

7. Get the victim to fresh air immediately; start artificial respiration if necessary (see page 42). Call the poison control center, doctor, or emergency room for further instructions.

8. Call the poison control center, doctor, or emergency room before attempting any first-aid treatment.

A
acetaminophen, 2
acetone, 2
acids
  ingestion, 4
  eye contamination, 6
  skin contamination, 5
  inhalation if mixed with bleach, 7
aerosols
  eye contamination, 6
  inhalation, 7
after-shave lotions
  less than ½ oz (15 ml), 1
  more than ½ oz (15 ml), 2
airplane glue, 8
alcohol
  ingestion, 2
  eye contamination, 6
alkalies
  ingestion, 4
  eye contamination, 6
  skin contamination, 5
  inhalation, 7
ammonia
  ingestion, 4
  eye contamination, 6
  inhalation, 7
amphetamines, 2
analgesics, 8

aniline dyes
  ingestion, 2
  inhalation, 7
  skin contamination, 5
antacids, 1
antibiotics
  less than 2 to 3 times total
    daily dose, 1
  more than 3 times total daily
    dose, 2
antidepressants
  tricyclic, 2
  others, 2
antifreeze (ethylene glycol)
  ingestion, 2
  eye contamination, 6
antihistamines, 2
antiseptics, 2
ant trap
  Kepone type, 1
  others, 2
aquarium products, 1
arsenic, 2
aspirin, 2
B
baby oil, 1
ball-point pen ink, 1
barbiturates
  short-acting, 8
  long-acting, 2

batteries
  dry cell (flashlight), 1
  mercury (hearing aid), 2
  wet cell (automobile), 4
benzene
  ingestion, 8
  inhalation, 7
  skin contamination, 5
birth-control pills, 1
bleaches
  liquid ingestion, 1
  solid ingestion, 4
  eye contamination, 6
  inhalation when mixed with
    acids or alkalies, 7
boric acid, 2
bromides, 2
bubble bath, 1
C
camphor, 2
candles, 1
caps for cap pistols
  less than one roll, 1
  more than one roll, 2
carbon monoxide, 7
carbon tetrachloride
  ingestion, 2
  inhalation, 7
  skin contamination, 5
chalk, 1

7

Poisons in the Workplace

A growing list
The number of toxic chemicals to which workers are exposed is rapidly increasing. In addition to such natural materials as lead, mercury, and silica, other materials taken from the earth, such as asbestos, radioactive ores, and petroleum products, can be toxic. And every year, we see an increasing number of synthetic, or artificially produced, chemicals.

Many people come into contact with poisonous or potentially harmful substances at work. Workers in hundreds of industries are exposed to toxic chemicals, dusts, and fumes. Contact with these substances can cause many kinds of occupational diseases.

Awareness of the dangers of working with chemicals has led to the establishment of government agencies that study the effects of chemicals and regulate their use by industry. The Occupational Safety and Health Administration and the National Institute of Occupational Safety and Health provide information on dangerous chemicals and establish regulations for their use. In particular, these agencies work to determine legal exposure limits for the chemicals that industry uses.

The existence of these government agencies doesn't guarantee you protection from harmful chemicals at work. Ideally, the toxic potential of a chemical should be determined before it's introduced into the workplace, but this isn't always possible since each year 700 to 1,000 new chemical compounds are introduced. While the government agencies are performing their tests, workers may be exposed to hazardous chemicals.

Routes of exposure

The majority of workplace poisons are inhaled; some are absorbed through the skin; only rarely today are workplace poisons swallowed. The few instances of accidentally ingested poisons usually result from a worker bringing food into a workroom—the chemical gets on the food and is swallowed with it.

Because most workplace poisons are either inhaled or absorbed by the skin, many work-related diseases caused by chemicals involve either the lungs or the skin. However, many toxic substances that enter the body through the lungs or skin get into the bloodstream and travel to other parts of the body, causing damage to other organs. Thus, the variety of work-related diseases is enormous.

Chronic poisonings

Some work-related diseases, such as dermatitis, show

Poisons in unlikely places
Factory workers aren't the only workers who risk exposure to dangerous substances; dangerous substances sometimes show up in unlikely places:
• Beauty salons. Hairdressers are routinely exposed to fumes from hair sprays and hair dyes. Constant inhalation of these fumes can lead to chronic lung disease and even to lung cancer.
• Hospital operating rooms. Doctors and nurses working in anesthetic-laden hospital operating rooms show an increased risk of cancer as a result of breathing the chemicals.

For more information

*Toxic Substances Control
Act Hotline
(800) 424-9065
Washington, D.C., area
only: (202) 554-1404
Answers questions on the
use of asbestos in schools,
polychlorinated biphenyls
(PCBs), and chlorofluoro-
carbons (CFCs). Also pro-
vides regulatory guidance
to industry on the Toxic
Substances Control Act. A
service of the Environmental Protection Agency.*

*National Pesticide
Information Clearinghouse
(800) 531-7790
TX only: (800) 292-7664
Responds to questions
about the health effects of
pesticides. A service of the
Environmental Protection
Agency.*

*Clearinghouse for
Occupational Safety and
Health Information
Technical Information
Branch
4676 Columbia Parkway
Cincinnati, OH 45226
(513) 684-8326
Provides technical informa-
tion support for the National
Institute for Occupational
Safety and Health research
programs and supplies in-
formation to others on re-
quest.*

Changes in skin color
*Skin contact with certain
chemicals such as silver
can cause changes in skin
color. Some chemicals
cause changes in skin color
when they get into the
bloodstream; consult a doctor if any area of your skin
changes color.*

up immediately or very soon after the first few exposures. However, most work-related diseases are
chronic poisonings—the results of long-term, repeated exposures—and develop only after many
years. In some cases, symptoms of disease may not
become evident for 20 years or more.

The most feared work-related disease is cancer,
caused by contact with cancer-causing substances
(carcinogens), but many other diseases can be caused
by chronic exposure to chemicals.

The most common occupational diseases that result from exposure to chemicals are:
• skin problems
• lung diseases caused by breathing dusts, fumes,
gases, and vapors
• cancer caused by repeated exposure to carcino-
genic substances.

Workers can also experience acute poisoning.

Skin problems
Dermatitis, or skin inflammation, is the most common
occupational disease. The first few exposures to a
chemical may cause no reaction, but with repeated
exposures the worker may become sensitized to the
chemical. Subsequent exposures, even to tiny quantities, may cause the person severe dermatitis. Photographic developers, dyes, oils, resins, and
plasticizers (chemicals added to rubber to make it
flexible) cause skin irritations in people who work
with them, but many other chemicals can cause skin
reactions.

Allergic reactions
In many cases, skin irritations are allergic reactions.
Many people suffer hives—reddish, circular welts that
form on the skin and itch and burn—from contact
with certain chemicals.

If you're troubled by hives or a persistent rash,
consult a doctor or dermatologist. You can be tested
to determine if you're allergic to a substance you
encounter at work.

Occupational acne
Some chemicals can cause what is known as chlor-
acne, or occupational acne. Among these chemicals
are certain oils, crude petroleum, coal tar, heavy tar
distillates, coal tar pitch, chlorinated hydrocarbons,
and some weed killers.

Special washing instructions

Garments that have come in contact with workplace chemicals should be washed by special laundering services. Don't take such garments home and throw them in with the family wash—to do so would expose your family and the environment to the chemicals.

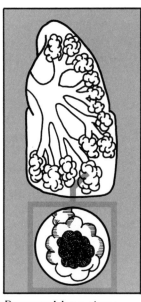

Damaged lung tissue

Prevention of skin exposure to chemicals

You can take several precautions to prevent skin exposure to chemicals:
• Gloves, sleeves, and aprons offer protection from contact with chemicals. Keep such garments clean and change them often; ideally, they should be washed every day.
• Wash all exposed skin—hands, face, arms—with soap and water frequently during the workday. Wash especially carefully before you eat, smoke, or leave work.
• Your doctor or dermatologist can recommend special ointments to use on your skin to prevent or treat dermatitis.
• If you develop a skin irritation that seems to be related to your work, consult your doctor or a dermatologist. Your problem may require a prescription drug.

Lung diseases

Workers in many industries are exposed to dusts, fumes, gases, and vapors. Such workers are susceptible to occupational lung diseases.

The best-known occupational lung diseases are caused by the inhalation of dusts. Such diseases are called pneumoconiosis. It's an occupational disease of miners, sandblasters, metal grinders, and stonecutters and is the result of repeated inhalation of dusts, including:
• iron oxides (such as rust and filings)
• silicates (talc, asbestos, and rock dusts)
• carbonates (coal dust).

Lung disease is caused by inhaled particles of dust that collect in the lungs. The irritation caused by these particles leads to tissue damage. As the disease progresses, the damaged areas enlarge, replacing more and more of the healthy, elastic tissue of the lungs. The disease can lead to lung cancer or to heart failure.

Lung disease symptoms include progressive shortness of breath, wheezing, chronic coughing, and frequent respiratory infections.

The inhalation of fumes, gases, and vapors can also result in an acute poisoning. Workers in mines, for example, risk exposure to hydrogen sulfide gas; workers in many industries are exposed to high levels of carbon monoxide.

Fishermen and tar
Tar has been shown to cause lip cancer in fishermen. Tar is used to keep fishing nets from rotting, and fishermen often put mending needles in their mouths while repairing nets, thus exposing their lips to tar.

Inhalation of various fumes causes a wide variety of illnesses. For example, many meat wrappers suffer so-called meat wrappers' asthma, which results from inhaling the fumes given off when the plastic used to wrap meat is cut with a hot wire.

Cancer
Many workers are exposed to cancer-causing chemicals (carcinogens). More than 30 chemical substances have been identified as causing cancer, among them:

- arsenic
- asbestos
- benzene
- chromium salts
- coke-oven by-products
- cutting oils
- mustard gas
- nickel
- polychlorinated biphenyl (PCB)
- soots and tars
- styrene butadiene
- synthetic rubber products
- vinyl chloride
- wood dust.

Different carcinogens affect different parts of the body. For example, workers in the plastics industry who handle vinyl chloride run a higher risk than the rest of the population of developing liver or brain cancer; workers in the rubber industry, in which benzidine (a suspected carcinogen) is used, run a greater risk of developing urinary bladder cancer.

Carcinogens are dangerous even in small amounts. Asbestos brought home on the clothing of asbestos workers has caused fatal cancers in members of the workers' families.

Skin cancers
Certain toxic substances, among them arsenic, tar, pitch, and oils, can cause skin cancers. Such skin cancers frequently begin as tumors or other skin growths. Consult a doctor immediately if you find any new growth on your skin or if any growth, such as a mole, changes shape or begins to bleed.

Latency period
Cancers develop slowly. Cancers of the liver, lung, or bladder, for example, may not appear until 20 to 30 years after exposure to a carcinogen.

This long period between exposure to a carcinogen and development of cancer is known as the latency period; because the latency period for most cancers is so long, a cancer's cause is often difficult to identify. By the time the cancer appears, the victim or the

Occupational safety precautions

- *Wear any required protective equipment such as gloves, goggles, aprons, masks, and protective clothing.*
- *Protective clothing should be laundered daily. Don't take it home to wash—use approved cleaning procedures.*
- *Air or gas masks should be used if necessary; they should be kept available for emergency use wherever dangerous substances are used.*
- *Wash all exposed skin—hands, face, arms—with soap and water frequently during the workday, especially before eating, smoking, and leaving work.*
- *Eye fountains and showers must be provided for immediate removal of spilled chemicals. Learn the locations of eye fountains and showers, and use them.*
- *In the event of a spill of a hazardous chemical, evacuate the room at once. Decontamination of spills is the job of specially trained personnel with adequate safety equipment.*
- *If you believe you're suffering from exposure to a toxic substance, report to your supervisor and seek medical assistance immediately.*

Any discomfort or body change can be an indication of a poisoning. Be particularly alert to:

- *skin rashes, eruptions, or swellings*
- *coughs, tightness in the chest, or difficult breathing*
- *difficult swallowing*
- *a cold that won't go away or repeated respiratory infections*
- *headaches, dizziness, or light-headedness*
- *eye irritations*
- *loss of appetite, fatigue, or nausea*
- *numbness in any body part.*

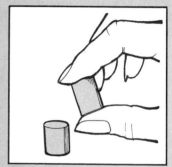

Ear molds

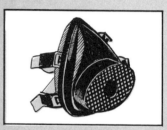

Respirator

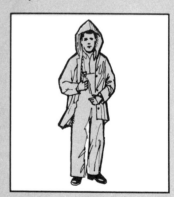

Protective clothing

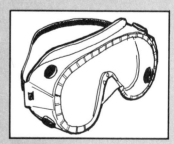

Safety glasses

Industrial-strength chemicals
The chemicals used in industries are stronger and more toxic that those available to the public—they're more dangerous and should be treated with extreme care.

victim's doctor may have difficulty remembering or finding the cause.

Acute poisonings

Your job may put you in danger of an acute poisoning. Examples of acute workplace poisonings are being overcome by toxic fumes or having a chemical spilled on your skin. Many workers suffer temporary headaches or eye irritation from accidental contact with chemicals.

Many chemicals can cause both acute and chronic poisonings. Pesticides and herbicides, for example, can cause dangerous acute poisonings and can also cause chronic poisonings.

Prevention of occupational poisonings

Learn as much as you can about the chemical or chemicals you work with. Information you should have includes:

• The chemical's name. Some industrial chemicals are called by trade names; try to find the generic (scientific) name of the chemical.

• The chemical's strength or concentration.

• The chemical's dangers, including possible chronic effects and their symptoms. In particular, you should determine whether or not the chemical is suspected of causing cancer.

Keep a record of your work history, including a list of all the chemicals you've been exposed to (length of exposures and dates).

If you work with chemicals, you should have a medical checkup every 6 months. Tell your doctor about the chemicals you work with, and share with your doctor whatever information you have about the chemicals. Since many doctors are unfamiliar with the symptoms of occupational diseases, you'll want one who knows about your work and its hazards.

8

Poisonous Gases

You breathe more than air, and some of what you breathe can harm you. Even if you don't smoke, you breathe in a frightening catalog of chemicals: the chemicals spewed into the air by industries, automobiles, and aerosol cans; and the chemical gases and vapors given off by various liquids.

Avoiding these chemicals isn't easy. Some, such as those created by industry and by automobiles, will remain with us until we decide to control the amount of pollution we permit in our world. Some, however, you can avoid.

Smelling danger

"If you can smell it, you're inhaling it." That simple rule applies to many, but not all, poisonous gases. If you're using an aerosol spray, and you can smell the product, you're inhaling it—and probably doing some damage to your lungs. The same applies to liquids, particularly certain household cleaners.

Unfortunately, you can't smell some gases, such as carbon monoxide; they have no odor. Thus, you can't depend on your nose to warn you of all dangerous gases.

Homemade poison gases

Confronted by stubborn stains on her bathroom tiles, Debbie decided to mix some ammonia into her tile cleaner. No sooner had she started scrubbing than her eyes began to bother her; then she found she was having trouble breathing. She got out of the bathroom fast and breathed deeply in front of an open window. She didn't feel better for several minutes.

By mixing common household cleansers, Debbie had created a poisonous gas—chloramine gas. The rule here is simple and important: never mix household cleansers. Doing so can create potentially deadly gases.

If you find yourself suffering symptoms from any cleanser, open a window and breathe in fresh air. Then open windows throughout your home to increase ventilation, and leave your home for a while. If you're still having difficulty breathing, go immediately to a hospital emergency room.

Dangerous mixtures
Mixing common household cleaners can create dangerous gases. The two most hazardous mixtures are:
• chlorine (bleach) plus ammonia, which creates chloramine gas
• chlorine (bleach) plus acid, which creates chlorine gas.
Products containing chlorine include household bleach, mildew removers, tile cleaners, and some powdered cleansers.
Household ammonia, glass cleaner, and floor and appliance detergents all may contain ammonia.
Toilet bowl cleaners contain acid.
Such mixtures create toxic gases that can irritate your eyes, nose, and throat and cause breathing difficulties. If you're exposed to enough of such a gas, you may be overcome by it. Inhaling such gases can cause injury requiring hospitalization; in extreme cases, inhaling these gases can be fatal.

Aerosol products
Hair sprays and other aerosols can alter the healthy functioning of lungs—and can do so very quickly. With just a 20-second direct exposure to a hair spray, you'll feel chest tightness and have difficulty breathing. Use such products only with adequate ventilation.

Adequate ventilation

Many products, among them oven cleaners, bug sprays, floor cleaners, and cleaning fluids, give off dangerous gases or vapors. Use such products only with adequate ventilation. If the weather's cold and you don't want to open a window, don't use these products. Always follow the label directions for protecting your eyes and skin, and avoid breathing the vapors.

Solvents

Solvents are cleaning agents that dissolve dirt and grime. All solvents are toxic; most can cause both acute and chronic poisonings. Furthermore, solvents are dangerous if spilled on the skin or into the eyes, if swallowed, or if inhaled.

Common household solvents include:
• carbon tetrachloride (used to clean metals, in dry cleaning, and to remove oil, grease, wax, and paint)
• benzene (used as a solvent for rubber, fats, greases, paints, and lacquers)
• methyl alcohol (used as a solvent and thinner for shellac, as a paint remover, and as a solvent for rubber cement)
• trichloroethylene (used as a metal degreaser, a solvent for oils and greases, and a paint remover)
• turpentine (used as a solvent and thinner for paint, varnish, and lacquer).

You should use these products outdoors if you can; if that isn't possible, open windows and doors and use a fan to increase ventilation. If you use solvents outdoors on a breezy day, work with the wind behind you so that the fumes blow away from you.

Breathing solvent fumes can cause several symptoms, such as headache, eye irritation, dizziness, visual disturbances, or nausea. In extreme cases, inhalation of these fumes can kill you.

If you experience any symptoms while using one of these products (or while one is being used nearby), get to fresh air immediately. If you continue to experience symptoms or have difficulty breathing, get to a hospital emergency room immediately.

Household cleansers
The chemicals in all household cleansers are dangerous. If you spill any cleanser on your skin, rinse the area in water for 15 minutes (see page 44); if you spill any into your eyes, rinse them for 15 to 20 minutes (see page 45). Then immediately call a poison control center, doctor, or emergency room for further instructions.

Carbon monoxide

Carbon monoxide gas results from the incomplete burning of organic substances, such as coal, wood, kerosene, paper, oil, cooking gas, or gasoline. Carbon monoxide is also in the exhaust of internal-combustion engines, including car engines.

Carbon monoxide gas

Common sources of carbon monoxide indoors are gas cooking ranges, hot water heaters, and driers; wood-burning or coal-burning stoves and fireplaces; oil burners; and kerosene heaters.

• Gas water heaters and driers and oil burners must have stacks that move the carbon monoxide outside.

• Wood-burning stoves and fireplaces must have chimneys that vent the poisonous gas outside.

• Unvented kerosene heaters spread carbon monoxide gas indoors. Always keep a window open slightly when you use a kerosene heater.

• Some gas cooking ranges have vents that draw poisonous gases outside. Otherwise, open a window when you use a gas stove or oven.

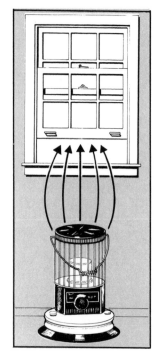

Carbon monoxide gas poisoning is the result of two factors:
• the presence of carbon monoxide in the air
• insufficient ventilation.

For example, a car engine left running in a closed garage can quickly produce a lethal dose of carbon monoxide.

Carbon monoxide gas is extremely poisonous. It doesn't irritate or damage the skin; instead, it kills by asphyxiation.

Inhaled carbon monoxide reacts with hemoglobin, the red blood cell pigment that carries oxygen to all parts of your body. Because carbon monoxide is attracted to the hemoglobin about 240 times as strongly as is oxygen, it takes the place of oxygen, causing oxygen starvation throughout the body's tissues. The brain suffers the most from lack of oxygen, and death occurs after only a short exposure.

Symptoms of carbon monoxide poisoning

Carbon monoxide gas is especially dangerous because you can't easily detect it: it has no smell, color, or taste. A victim may die with no awareness of carbon monoxide poisoning.

Carbon monoxide poisoning produces these early symptoms: headache, dizziness, drowsiness, weakness, nausea (with possible vomiting), rapid breathing, and flushed skin. As the level of carbon monoxide in the blood increases, the victim may experience confusion, impaired judgment, dulled sensation, clumsiness, and dimness of vision. Loss of consciousness quickly follows.

First aid for carbon monoxide poisoning

First-aid procedures for carbon monoxide poisoning are very much like those for all inhaled poisons (see page 43). Follow these steps:

1. Call for help and get the victim to fresh air immediately.

• If you can't move the victim, open all windows and doors.

• If possible, shut off the source of the gas.

• Loosen any tight clothing on the victim.

2. If the victim isn't breathing or is breathing irregularly, open his airway and begin artificial respiration immediately (see page 42).

Don't stop giving artificial respiration until the victim is breathing well or help arrives.

3. Keep the victim warm and quiet to help prevent shock.

Prevention of carbon monoxide poisoning

Proper ventilation is the most important step in preventing carbon monoxide poisoning. Carbon monoxide poisoning is a hazard whenever you light a flame in a poorly ventilated place.

Cars

• Don't sit in the car in a closed garage and run the engine. Even with the garage door open, don't run the engine for more than a minute or two.

• Open station-wagon tailgate windows or hatchback doors pull in carbon monoxide; always open other windows to produce a safe airflow.

• Don't sit in a parked car with the engine running for more than a few minutes unless the windows are open.

Furnaces, stoves, heaters

• Carbon monoxide can be generated by wood, coal, and charcoal fires and by faulty oil burners.

• Gas heaters should be provided with vents.

• Furnaces and automatic exhausts should be checked regularly to make certain they're in good working order. If you light a heater, stove, or furnace after a long period of disuse, check at once to see that it's working properly and that the flue or chimney is clear.

• All furnaces, stoves, and heaters should be vented to the outside. Make certain that venting pipes, flues, and chimneys are free of soot or other obstructions (such as bird nests). Inspect all flues and chimneys at least once a year. Replace or repair corroded sections or cracked linings.

• Never use charcoal grills or hibachis in enclosed areas without adequate ventilation.

• Never use unvented equipment that burns charcoal as a source of heat in a tent, trailer, camper, car, boat, or home.

• Never use a kerosene space heater without opening a window.

• Never use a kitchen's gas stove as a heater.

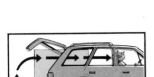

Protect yourself
Airflow through an open tailgate window pulls exhaust gases, including carbon monoxide, into a car.

Lawnmowers
Don't run a lawnmower— or tune one up—in a closed garage or shed.

Tiny amounts are deadly
Breathing air that contains as little as 0.1% carbon monoxide by volume can be fatal; a concentration of about 1% can cause death within a few minutes. Car exhaust contains 1% to 7% carbon monoxide.

9

Poisonous Plants

Plants and people

Plants are vital to our existence. They help provide the oxygen we breathe and are an essential food source. Besides giving us grains, fruits, and vegetables, plants offer us wood, fibers, oils, latex, pigments, resins, and drugs; coal and petroleum are of plant origin. Plants feed us and provide us with shelter and the raw materials from which countless other products are made.

The vast majority of plants are either edible or harmless if swallowed. Most of those that are poisonous are only mildly poisonous; a few are extremely poisonous. Some plants are poisonous only at certain stages of their growth. Young pokeweed, for example, is eaten as a vegetable green, but older pokeweed plants are poisonous. In many cases only part of a plant is poisonous. The leaf blades of rhubarb are poisonous; the stalks aren't. Some plants are always poisonous and are poisonous in every part; some that are poisonous to humans aren't poisonous to animals. Birds thrive on berries that are poisonous to humans, and a variety of mushroom that rabbits nibble on without ill effect may quickly kill a human.

You don't need to travel to rural areas or distant jungles to find poisonous plants: there may be some in your backyard. Perhaps there's one hanging in your kitchen window and another on a shelf in the living room. Such familiar plants as daffodils, philodendrons, hyacinths, oleander, and lily of the valley are poisonous.

You wouldn't eat one of these plants, but children might—and do. Every year, many thousands of children suffer from plant poisoning, and the ingestion of plant materials by children is a leading cause of visits or calls to a poison control center. Most of the children poisoned by plants don't need to be hospitalized, but some are severely—even fatally—injured. Often, only very small amounts of the plant are involved.

The appeal of plants

Toddlers are the most frequent victims of plant poisonings. Whether to satisfy curiosity or to relieve the sensations of teething, they put anything within reach into their mouths. Plants are particularly appealing: they have pretty colors, nice smells, and, in many cases, attractive, bite-size berries. They look like food.

Prevention of plant poisoning

To make your home safe for children, you must eliminate the danger of plant poisoning.

• Keep all plants out of the reach of young children. Even nonpoisonous plants can be harmful: many are sprayed with insecticides.

• Store bulbs and seeds out of sight and reach.

• Identify the poisonous plants in your home and neighborhood. Check the list of poisonous plants (see page 92). If you aren't sure about a plant, take it or a piece of it to a plant store or nursery for positive identification. If you know the name of the plant but it doesn't appear on the list, call a botanical society or poison control center.

• Label all indoor and outdoor plants. Learning plant names can be fun—and educational—and knowing the names of your plants can provide vital information in the event of an accidental poisoning. Plant stores, nurseries, and botanical societies can all help identify plants.

• Put a poison warning label, such as a "Mr. Yuk" sticker, on poisonous indoor plants. Do this only if you're using such warning labels to identify other poisons, and remember that this is an activity to perform with your child. Make it clear that these plants are as dangerous as the other things you've labeled with the warning labels.

• Don't buy poisonous plants. Before buying a plant, ask the salesclerk if it's poisonous. If the salesclerk isn't sure, get the name of the plant, and check it yourself. Don't rely on the knowledge of salesclerks in stores that don't specialize in selling plants.

• Supervise children closely when they're playing near plants. Bits and pieces of plants sometimes make their way into children's games. Teach your children never to use plants as play foods. Be alert: Retrieving a baseball can bring a child into contact with unknown plants or poison ivy, oak, or sumac.

• Teach your children never to eat any part of any plant without your approval. This applies both indoors and outdoors. Children must be taught not to eat anything they pick up outside. Some of the most attractive fruits and berries are the most poisonous, and even familiar plants can present dangers. Acorns, for example, can cause constipation, bloody stools, and gradual kidney damage if enough are eaten. It takes a large amount for poisoning, but children shouldn't be permitted to chew on acorns—or any other plant parts.

• Check your houseplants periodically. Look for telltale clues: torn or missing leaves, broken branches, missing berries. If you find such indications of a child's handiwork, relocate the plant even if it isn't poisonous.

• Get rid of poisonous plants. You may decide to avoid all risk by getting rid of the poisonous plants in and around your home. You don't need to destroy the plants. If some of your favorite plants are poisonous, give them to a friend or neighbor to care for until your children are older. You don't have to do without plants: many plants are nonpoisonous (see page 93).

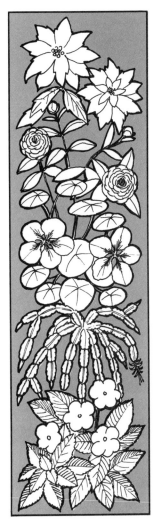

Safe plants:
Poinsettia
Camellia
Nasturtium
Christmas cactus
Impatiens

Poisonous plants: poisonous parts and symptoms

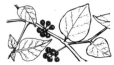

Black nightshade *(Solanum nigrum)*

☠ Leaves and unripe fruit

Symptoms usually appear after a few hours and include a scratchy or burning sensation in the throat, nausea, vomiting, stomach pain, diarrhea, mental confusion, weakness, difficulty breathing, and fever.

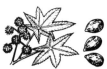

Castor bean *(Ricinus communis)*

☠ All parts, especially seeds (if chewed; if swallowed whole, the hard seed coat prevents absorption and poisoning)

Symptoms usually develop after several hours and include a burning sensation in the mouth and throat, severe and bloody diarrhea (this plant is the source of castor oil, a cathartic), nausea, vomiting, severe stomach cramps, blurred vision, and convulsions. Two to four well-chewed seeds can be fatal to a child.

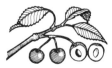

Cherries, wild and cultivated *(Prunus)*

☠ Pits and leaves

Shortness of breath; vocal cord paralysis; muscle twitching; weakness; seizures; altered state of awareness, including unconsciousness; stupor; coma. The pits contain a substance that, when eaten, releases cyanide.

Daphne, spurge laurel *(Daphne mezereum)*

☠ All parts, especially the berries

Swelling and blistering of lips, increased salivation and difficulty swallowing, stomach pain, vomiting, bloody diarrhea, altered state of awareness, weakness, and convulsions. Just a few berries can be fatal to a child.

Dumb cane, dieffenbachia *(Dieffenbachia)*

☠ All parts, including sap

Blistering and burning of mouth and tongue with swelling of tongue and throat and difficulty swallowing, nausea, vomiting, diarrhea, excessive salivation. Also causes vocal cord paralysis, which makes speech unintelligible—hence the name dumb cane.

Foxglove *(Digitalis purpurea)*

☠ All parts

Nausea, vomiting, diarrhea, stomach pain, severe headache, loss of appetite, irregular heartbeat and pulse, tremors, convulsions. This plant is a source of the drug digitalis, and large amounts of it cause dangerously irregular heartbeat and pulse.

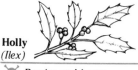

Holly *(Ilex)*

☠ Berries and leaves

Nausea, vomiting, diarrhea, inflammation and numbing sensation in the mouth, drowsiness, altered state of awareness.

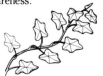

Ivy, English ivy, Boston ivy, and others *(Hedera)*

☠ All parts

Nausea, vomiting, diarrhea, difficulty breathing, abdominal pain, excessive salivation, coma, skin irritation.

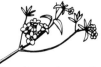

Jasmine, jessamine, yellow jessamine *(Gelsemium sempervirens)*

☠ All parts

Headache, dizziness, drooping eyelids, profuse sweating, muscular weakness, convulsions, difficulty breathing. Children are frequently poisoned by sucking on the flowers.

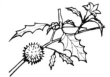

Jimsonweed, thorn apple, stinkweed *(Datura stramonium)*

☠ All parts, but especially seeds

Intense thirst and dry mouth; dilated pupils; dry, hot, flushed skin; headache; rapid, weak pulse; visual difficulty; fever; hallucinations; disorientation; urinary retention and decreased bowel activity; high blood pressure; delirium, convulsions, coma. Handling the leaves and then rubbing your eyes can cause dilation of pupils.

Lily of the valley *(Convallaria majalis)*

 All parts

Slow or irregular heartbeat, nausea. Dizziness and vomiting may occur in 1 to 2 hours if large quantities are eaten.

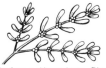

Mistletoe (American: *Phoradendron flavescens;* European: *Viscum album*)

 Stems, leaves, berries

Severe nausea, vomiting, and diarrhea; stomach cramps; difficulty breathing and slow pulse; delirium; hallucinations; coma. The berries are particularly dangerous, and several children have died after eating them. Tea brewed from the berries has also caused death.

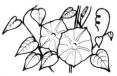

Morning glory, heavenly blue, pearly gates, flying saucers *(Ipomoea)*

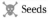 Seeds

Nausea, vomiting, distortion of time and space, hallucinations. From 50 to 200 powdered seeds can produce symptoms similar to those of LSD.

Oleander *(Nerium oleander)*

All parts

Nausea, severe vomiting, stomach pain, dizziness, altered state of awareness, slow or irregular pulse, dilated pupils, bloody diarrhea, drowsiness, slow respirations. One leaf can kill an adult.

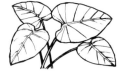

Philodendron *(Philodendron)*

All parts

Intense burning of mucous membranes with swelling of tongue, lips, mouth, and throat; nausea, vomiting, diarrhea; excessive salivation.

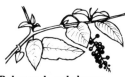

Pokeweed, pokeberry, scoke, inkberry *(Phytolacca americana)*

All parts, especially roots

Burning and bitter taste in mouth, persistent vomiting, stomach cramps, diarrhea, difficulty breathing, weakness, tremors, visual disturbances, convulsions. Poisonings are frequently the result of mistaking the roots for horseradish or parsnips.

Rhododendron *(Rhododendron)*

All parts

Increased salivation, vomiting, convulsions, tearing eyes and a discharge from the nose, difficulty breathing and slowing of pulse, convulsions, muscle weakness progressing to paralysis. Poisonings have occured from eating honey made from the plant's nectar.

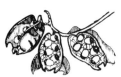

Rosary pea or bean, jequirity bean, prayer bead, Indian licorice, crab eye, precatory bean *(Abrus precatorius)*

Seeds or beans (if chewed; if swallowed whole, the hard seed coat prevents absorption and poisoning)

Symptoms usually appear after several hours and include mouth irritations; nausea; vomiting; severe diarrhea; weakness; cold, clammy skin with perspiration; weak, rapid pulse; tremors. One well-chewed bean can be fatal.

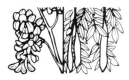

Wisteria *(Wisteria)*

All parts, especially seeds and pods

Burning in mouth and throat, nausea, vomiting, stomach pain, diarrhea.

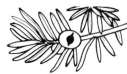

Yew *(Taxus)*

All parts

Symptoms appear after a short delay and include dizziness, dry mouth, nausea, vomiting, diarrhea, stomach pain, difficulty breathing, muscle weakness, slow pulse, and coma. A rash may appear, and the victim's face may become pale and the lips bluish. The red berries are attractive to children.

The most dangerous plants

Dumb cane and philodendron are responsible for more cases of distress (although not serious poisoning) in young children than all other plants combined. Pay special attention to these plants.

• Teach children not to chew on beans or seeds. Poisonous beans or seeds can enter your home as beadwork jewelry or inside rattles and maracas. Rosary, or jequirity, beans are commonly used in such items. The fact that the beans are part of a beadwork necklace or are inside a rattle doesn't make them any less poisonous. Any articles made of or containing unknown beans should be kept away from children.

Fruit seeds can also be dangerous if eaten in large amounts. The seeds or pits of apples, pears, peaches, plums, apricots, and wild cherries contain cyanide.

• Don't forget vegetable garden plants. Three common vegetable garden plants—tomatoes, potatoes, and rhubarb—can be poisonous. The leaves and stems of tomato plants contain a dangerous chemical called solanine. Solanine is also present in green potatoes and potato vines, leaves, and tubercles. In large enough amounts, solanine can cause abdominal pain, jaundice, vomiting, and diarrhea.

The leaf blades (not the stalks) of rhubarb contain a poisonous acid that can cause intense burning and irritation of the mouth and throat.

• Don't assume a plant isn't poisonous because birds or other animals eat it.

• Don't make homemade "medicines" or teas from plants.

Symptoms and first-aid treatment for plant poisoning

The most common symptoms of plant poisoning include nausea, vomiting, diarrhea, and digestive upset (including severe stomachache); burning and irritation of the mouth, tongue, and throat; difficulty breathing; nervous excitement; an altered state of awareness, including unconsciousness; mental confusion (some plants cause hallucinations); an irregular heartbeat and pulse; sweating; excessive salivation; convulsions; dilated or constricted pupils; and coma. Greenish bowel movements can be caused by the ingestion of poisonous or nonpoisonous plants.

These aren't the only possible symptoms of plant poisoning, and the presence of one or more of these symptoms doesn't necessarily mean that a child (or anyone else) has been poisoned by a plant. Many other things can cause these symptoms, and some of these symptoms, such as diarrhea, can be the result of common maladies.

Call a poison control center immediately in the

Other precautions

Pick up and discard fallen leaves and berries, and keep children away from the water used in plant vases. With some plants, such as oleander and lily of the valley, this water can become poisonous.

Plants and pets

Poison control centers receive frequent calls from distressed pet owners concerning animals that have eaten plants. What's dangerous to a human isn't necessarily dangerous to an animal; in most cases, there's nothing to fear if your family dog devours the better part of a bush.

event of plant poisoning. If the victim has serious symptoms, such as an irregular heartbeat or difficulty breathing, also call an ambulance.

If you suspect that your child has put any part of a poisonous plant—or an unknown plant—into his or her mouth, call a poison control center immediately, whether or not symptoms are present. In many cases, the symptoms of plant poisoning don't appear for several hours. Be ready to identify the plant. If you don't know the plant's name, get a piece of it. A sample of the plant, with flowers and seeds if possible, is important for positive identification if specific treatment is required. If you can't locate the plant, save the plant particles from stool or vomit.

Most victims of plant poisonings don't require medical treatment. You may be instructed simply to observe the victim, to give milk or water, to induce vomiting with ipecac syrup, or to bring the victim in for immediate emergency medical attention. If medical help isn't readily available, you should make the victim vomit. Follow the instructions on page 41.

Poisonous plants and symptoms

Twenty of the most common poisonous plants are listed and illustrated on pages 60 and 61. (You'll find a more complete list, as well as a list of nonpoisonous plants, on pages 92 and 93.) The plants are listed alphabetically by their common names; alternate names and Latin names are also given. Remember that not all of the symptoms may occur, and some may be more or less severe.

You'll see that the poisoning symptoms for many of these plants are very similar. That's why identification of the plant is so important in a poisoning emergency. A piece of the plant or particles from vomit or stool will help identify the plant.

Mushrooms

The mushrooms you buy in food stores are delicious; those you find in the woods are poisonous. This rule is simple, but every year people pick wild mushrooms, eat them, and get sick. Many die.

The attractions of wild mushrooms are several. Connoisseurs prize them for their unique, woodsy flavors. Back-to-nature disciples extol their healthful qualities. And they're free—all you have to do is go out and pick them.

Not all wild mushrooms are poisonous, of course, but telling the difference between poisonous and non-

Mushroom lore
*Contrary to popular folk-
lore, a silver spoon or coin
put in a pan with cooking
mushrooms won't turn
black if the mushrooms are
poisonous. Poisonous mushrooms won't darken if
soaked in water; nor will
they become milky if
soaked in vinegar. Nibble
marks on a mushroom in-
dicate only that a small animal has been eating at
it—they don't mean the
mushroom is safe for hu-
mans. The animal may
well have died after eating
the mushrooms, and some
mushrooms deadly to hu-
mans don't harm animals.*

poisonous mushrooms requires a mycologist—a mushroom expert—and even they sometimes make errors because mushrooms are tricky. Some are always poisonous; some are poisonous only occasionally or at certain stages of growth. Some are poisonous when eaten raw, but no amount of cooking will destroy the poisons in mushrooms. In some cases, the fumes coming from a pot in which mushrooms are being cooked are poisonous. Poisonous mushrooms grow in the same areas as nonpoisonous mushrooms, and many poisonous kinds look exactly like nonpoisonous kinds. Nonpoisonous mushrooms can be contaminated by toxic wastes or pesticides. Finally, the poisons in mushrooms have different effects on different people. The fact that someone else has eaten a particular kind of mushroom without ill effect doesn't necessarily mean that it's safe for you to eat.

The poisonous mushrooms most frequently encountered in this country are those of the genus *Amanita,* including *Amanita muscaria* and *Amanita phalloides.* The latter is the most dangerous mushroom in the world. Its nicknames are indicative: destroying angel and death cup. Cooking, freezing, or drying will neither destroy nor neutralize the poisons. The mortality for those who eat them is frightening: 50% to 90% if untreated; 22% if treated.

Symptoms and first-aid treatment of mushroom poisoning

The first symptoms of mushroom poisoning are usually nausea, vomiting, cramps, and diarrhea. If these symptoms develop more than 6 hours after the mushroom was eaten, the mushroom was probably highly toxic. Some mushrooms, particularly *Amanita phalloides,* contain slow-acting poisons. The victim may experience terrible stomach pain and then feel fine for 6 to 8 days. By then, the poisons in the mushroom will have caused serious damage to the victim's kidneys and liver.

If you have any reason to believe that you or someone else has eaten a poisonous mushroom, call a poison control center, doctor, or emergency room immediately.

You may be instructed to make the victim vomit with ipecac syrup (see page 40). Antidotes are available for many mushroom poisons, but because of the many kinds of poisonous mushrooms, there are many different treatments. It's important to give the medical personnel a specimen of the mushroom. If possible, it should be freshly picked and should include the stem, cap, and base. Keep it loosely wrapped in paper, not plastic.

Poisonous mushrooms and symptoms

The poisonous mushrooms illustrated here are the two most commonly encountered in the United States. These illustrations aren't for purposes of identification. Only an expert mycologist can distinguish poisonous from nonpoisonous mushrooms.

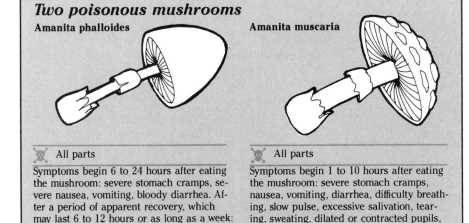

Two poisonous mushrooms

Amanita phalloides

Amanita muscaria

☠ All parts

Symptoms begin 6 to 24 hours after eating the mushroom: severe stomach cramps, severe nausea, vomiting, bloody diarrhea. After a period of apparent recovery, which may last 6 to 12 hours or as long as a week: decreased urination, headache, confusion, convulsions, hallucinations, coma.

☠ All parts

Symptoms begin 1 to 10 hours after eating the mushroom: severe stomach cramps, nausea, vomiting, diarrhea, difficulty breathing, slow pulse, excessive salivation, tearing, sweating, dilated or contracted pupils, hallucinations, delirium, muscle tremors, coma.

Poison ivy, poison oak, poison sumac

In addition to those plants that are poisonous when eaten, several plants are poisonous to the touch. You're probably familiar with the three best known of these: poison ivy, poison oak, and poison sumac.

Poison ivy, oak, and sumac are three closely related members of the *Rhus* genus. The sap of all three contains a resin known as urushiol. Skin contact with urushiol causes an allergic reaction known as contact dermatitis in many people. Although the urushiols of the three plants aren't identical, they're sufficiently similar for a person allergic to one to react to all three.

The allergic response to these three plants varies from person to person. Some people experience mild itching and slight inflammation of the affected area, and others suffer severe burning and itching followed by formation of watery blisters that ooze and then

Related offenders

If you're allergic to poison ivy, oak, and sumac, you may also be allergic to other related plants. Among these are cashews, pistachios, mangos, and Chinese or Japanese lacquer trees. Some people experience outbreaks from the oil of cashew shells; some experience allergic reactions after handling wooden and lacquered items made in China and Japan. (The name urushiol *comes from a Japanese word meaning "lacquer.")*

66

Dangerous smoke

Urushiol can also be carried in smoke from burning plants. Branches of these plants are sometimes accidentally gathered for firewood, and people trying to rid their yards of the plants sometimes burn them. The smoke given off by these plants is particularly dangerous because it can enter the nasal passages, throat, and lungs of anyone breathing it.

crust over. Not everyone will have a reaction, but 7 of 10 Americans are allergic to these plants and will develop contact dermatitis if exposed to large enough doses of urushiol; 5 of 10 Americans develop dermatitis if exposed to much smaller doses.

The allergic reaction is most common in adults and rare in children. This is because children have had fewer opportunities to come in contact with the plants, and the allergic reaction doesn't usually develop after the first exposure. Indeed, the first time you come in contact with poison ivy, oak, or sumac, you probably won't suffer at all. You may not even realize you've come in contact with the plant, or if you know you have, you may be led to believe you're not sensitive to it.

You don't have to touch a plant to come in contact with urushiol because urushiol is easily transferred from one object or person to another. Anything that comes in contact with the plant—clothing, gardening tools, pets, sports equipment—can pick up the urushiol and pass it to someone or something else. And urushiol can remain active for as long as a year. Anything that may have come in contact with the plant must be washed thoroughly.

Symptoms and treatment of poison ivy, oak, or sumac poisoning

After contact, itching and burning may appear in a matter of hours or days but usually develop within 24 to 48 hours in a sensitized person. The skin that has touched the plant or the urushiol becomes reddened, then watery blisters appear. There is also usually itching, burning, and swelling. The rash is worst after about 5 days and then gradually improves within a week or two even without treatment. The blisters break, and the oozing sores begin to crust over and disappear.

The first and most essential part of treatment is to wash the affected area with soap and cold water. This must be done immediately. Use yellow laundry soap if available and lather several times, rinsing the area in running water after each sudsing. Don't scrub with a brush. If you're in the woods, the water of a running stream will do the job. Any clothing that might have come in contact with the urushiol must be washed and rewashed.

Having washed off the urushiol, you'll require little or no further treatment of mild cases of rash. The

Poison ivy

The old saying "leaflets three, let it be" (or "leaves of three, quickly flee") is sound advice. Poison ivy has slightly glossy green leaves that grow in groups of three. The leaves may be notched or smooth, but they always grow in clusters of three—one at the end of the stalk, the other two opposite each other. In the early fall, the leaves may turn an attractive red. Although it usually grows as a vine, poison ivy can grow as a low shrub, especially along fences or stone walls or in fields. There may be waxy, yellow-green flowers and greenish berries with markings that make them look like a peeled orange. Recognizing these berries can help you identify the plants in late fall, winter, and early spring when the leaves aren't present. Although it's most common in the eastern and central states, poison ivy grows throughout the United States.

Poison oak

The leaves of poison oak also grow in groups of three. The resemblance of these leaves to oak leaves gives the plant its name. Because they're covered with fine hairs, the undersides of the leaves are a much lighter green than the tops. There may be clusters of greenish or creamy white berries, but not all plants bear fruit. Poison oak usually grows as a low shrub and is most common on the west coast from Mexico to British Columbia.

Poison sumac

Poison sumac has 7 to 13 leaves arranged in pairs with a single leaf at the end of the stem. The leaves are long and smooth. In the spring, they're bright orange and velvetlike; they later become dark green and glossy on the upper surface and light green on the lower. Early in the fall, they become reddish orange. Poison sumac can be distinguished from nonpoisonous sumacs by its drooping clusters of green berries; nonpoisonous sumacs have red, upright berry clusters. Poison sumac grows as a tree, usually 5 or 6 feet high, although some grow to 25 feet. It's found in swampy areas throughout the eastern United States.

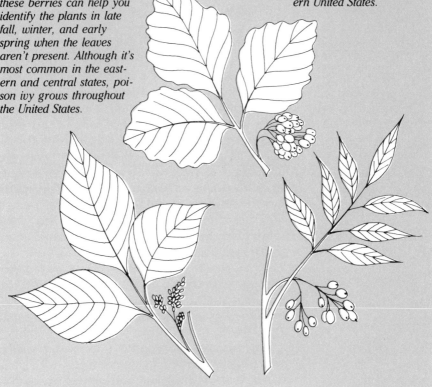

Don't scratch

Contrary to popular belief, scratching and breaking the blisters won't cause the rash to spread. There's no urushiol in the blister fluid. However, you should avoid scratching and even touching the affected areas. If the urushiol hasn't been completely washed off the skin, touching the affected areas and then another part of the body can transfer the urushiol—and the rash. The rash can't be passed from person to person unless the urushiol hasn't been washed off the skin of the affected person. You should also avoid scratching because scratching the rash may introduce bacteria into the sores, causing an infection.

sores will heal on their own. You can relieve the itching and burning by applying compresses soaked in cool water or Burow's solution. A calamine lotion or other preparation with calamine in it, such as Caladryl, spread over the rash will help dry the area while also relieving the itching and burning.

If you know you're highly sensitive to these plants, you should see your doctor immediately if you come in contact with one of them. If you suffer frequent or severe outbreaks, ask your doctor about desensitization. Desensitization is also a good idea for people who work outdoors.

Identifying poison ivy, poison oak, and poison sumac

The best way to prevent contact dermatitis from these plants is to learn how to recognize them and stay away from them. Fortunately, this isn't difficult.

To avoid contact with these plants:
• Teach children to identify and avoid these plants.
• Always wear long sleeves, long pants, and gloves when working outdoors where these plants are known to exist or when hiking in unfamiliar woods.
• Thoroughly wash any article of clothing that comes in contact with one of these plants.
• Remember that although animals don't usually react to urushiol, they can carry it on their fur. If you think the wanderings of your family pet may have brought it in contact with one of these plants, give it a bath.

If you find these plants growing in your backyard, you'll want to get rid of them. The U.S. Department of Agriculture recommends the use of herbicides (chemical weed killers). Follow the directions carefully. These chemicals are poisons and can do harm to both valuable vegetation and people. They should be carefully sprayed or even painted on the leaves of the plants. Store any leftover herbicide in a locked cabinet, and dispose of empty containers according to the directions on the container.

The plants can also be destroyed by grubbing (digging up their roots). This can be accomplished only when the ground is thoroughly wet. If the ground is dry, the roots will break off in the ground and sprout again later.

Take care not to touch the plants when working with them. Don't burn the uprooted plants, and don't bundle them up and leave them for the garbage man. They should be buried.

10 Poisonous Animals and Insects

The effects of venoms
Injected into the skin of a human, venoms produce symptoms that range from itching and swelling to paralysis and, in rare cases, death. The effects of venoms vary according to several factors, including:
• *how much venom is injected*
• *the age and size of the victim—because of their small size, children are more severely injured by venoms than are adults*
• *the amount of protective clothing the victim is wearing*
• *where the venom is injected into the victim, the depth of the bite (and the number of bites), and how long it takes for the venom to be absorbed into the victim's bloodstream*
• *how long it takes for the victim to receive medical care*
• *the victim's sensitivity to the venom*
• *the kind of first aid and medical care that the victim receives.*

Copperheads
Copperheads have copper-colored heads. Their bodies, too, are coppery or pale pink with darker crossbands forming hourglass shapes. Rarely more than 3 feet long, they can be found in the eastern United States from New England to Florida and west to Texas.

Venoms are poisonous substances produced by various snakes, lizards, spiders, scorpions, insects, and other animals. When these animals bite or sting, they inject their venom. Some animals use their venom only for self-defense; some use their venom to paralyze or kill prey. Some, particularly snakes, have venoms that aid in the digestion of prey.

Poisonous snakes

Poisonous snakes have fangs—long, hollow or grooved teeth usually located on the upper jaw. When the snake bites it prey, venom flows from poison glands through or over the fangs and into the prey.

Snake venom is a complex substance and contains various toxins. Some snake venom is primarily hemotoxic—poisonous to the blood—and destroys blood cells. Some is primarily neurotoxic—poisonous to the nerves—and produces paralysis. Venoms may also contain substances that either promote or inhibit blood coagulation. Venoms vary greatly with the species of snake, the snake's age, and even its geographical location.

An antivenin is an antidote to snake venom. Antivenins exist for all the dangerous snake venoms. Because venoms are different, antivenins are different, and identification of the snake can be important for effective treatment of a snakebite.

Four types of poisonous snake live in the United States: rattlesnakes, copperheads, water moccasins, and coral snakes. Learning to recognize these snakes will help you avoid them and describe them in the event of a snakebite.

Like all poisonous snakes, those found in this country have fangs. A snake without fangs can be considered harmless; a snake with fangs is probably poisonous.

Rattlesnakes, copperheads, and water moccasins are called pit vipers because they have a small, deep pit between the nostril and eye on each side of the head. These pits are heat detectors that enable the snake to sense the warmth given off by other animals.

Pit vipers can also be identified by their flattened, triangular heads and slitlike eyes (these eyes are also

Rattlesnakes

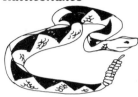

Rattlesnakes have rattles; no other snakes have them, and they're easy to spot. The rattles are interlocking segments of hollow scales that form a series of rings at the end of the snake's tail. When the snake shakes its tail—usually just before striking—the segments rattle against one another to produce a whirring noise.

Rattlesnakes are found in most of the 48 continental states, particularly in the drier regions of the south and west. They vary greatly in size and coloration.

Water moccasins, or cottonmouths

Water moccasins, also known as cottonmouths, are particularly dangerous because they rarely move away if disturbed. However, they give a kind of warning before striking: they gape widely, displaying the inside of their mouths, which are white— hence the name cottonmouth.

Usually just over 3 feet long, they have black, olive, or brown bodies. They're found in the southeastern United States, mainly in the swamplands of Mississippi and Florida.

present in some nonpoisonous snakes). Coral snakes have bullet-shaped heads and round eyes, but they don't have pits.

Prevention of snakebites

If you live in or visit a snake-inhabited area, you should observe certain precautions. Some of these precautions are intended to warn snakes of your approach. Snakes are deaf to sounds in the air, but their inner ears pick up vibrations from the ground, such as footfalls. Snakes are also very short-sighted.

• Watch where you're going. When moving through an area where there may be snakes, pay close attention to where you step and where you place your hands. Never put either your feet or your hands where you can't see them. If you must walk through tall grass or bushes, poke the clumps ahead with a stick to alert any snakes to your approach. Don't reach above your head where you can't see, or put your hands into crevices.

• Wear heavy, leather, high-top shoes or boots and loose-fitting long pants. The cuffs of the pants should reach over the tops of the shoes. If a snake strikes, it may snag its fangs in your pants rather than your skin.

• When camping outdoors, avoid areas near rocks, logs, burrows, or caves.

• Always wear heavy gloves when cleaning up debris, particularly logs or old lumber. Before picking up a log or board, use a stick or crowbar to raise one end so you can see if it's safe to pick up.

Symptoms and first-aid treatment of snakebite

The bite of a snake can be swift and almost gentle or it can be painful; it can feel like the prick of a hypodermic needle or like a sharp stab. The fangs produce puncture marks, usually twin slits that may ooze venom mixed with blood.

The first symptom of a pit viper bite usually appears within 3 to 5 minutes: burning, often excruciating pain at the site of the injury. Swelling and discoloration begin within 10 minutes. The swelling increases rapidly; an arm can swell to twice its normal size within an hour. The victim may experience blurred or dimmed vision, weakness, drowsiness, nausea, vomiting, and excessive salivation and sweating. Other symptoms, including numbness of the tongue and mouth, difficult breathing, and shock, may de-

Coral snakes

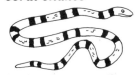

Coral snakes are easily identified by their small, bullet-shaped black heads and small, round black eyes. Their slender bodies have a waxy, shiny appearance and are marked with bands of contrasting colors—red, black, and yellow. Several nonpoisonous snakes have similarly banded bodies. The rule is that the red bands are bordered by black bands on harmless snakes; on coral snakes, the red bands are bordered by yellow bands. Don't take the time to sort this out if you're confronted by a snake.

Don't apply a tourniquet

A constricting band isn't a tourniquet. A tourniquet is tied so tightly that deep circulation is cut off; in the case of a snakebite, this can do more harm to a limb than the venom. A rule to remember: Applying a tourniquet results in the loss of that limb.

Sucking venom

Don't try to suck the venom from the wound. Regardless of what you've seen in movies, this is more likely to do harm than good. Very little venom remains at the site of the wound, and, at best, sucking will remove only 20% of the poison injected by the snake.

velop within hours of the bite.

Coral snake venom may cause no immediate symptoms except for slight burning, prickling, or mild swelling at the site of the bite. Other symptoms may not develop for several hours, but they progress rapidly and include weakness, drooping eyelids, slurred speech, increased salivation, sweating, nausea, and vomiting. Paralysis, difficult breathing, convulsions, and shock follow.

A poisonous snakebite is a medical emergency, but even if the bite is fairly serious, you have time— usually as long as several hours—to get professional help before the injury becomes life-threatening.

- Keep the victim calm and get medical help immediately.
- Make the victim lie down. If the victim must be moved, he or she should be carried. It's best for one person to stay with the victim while another goes for help.
- Keep the bitten area horizontal, below the level of the victim's heart, and wash the wound with soap and water.
- Try to identify the snake. Do this only after the victim is on the way to a hospital or a doctor has been summoned. Don't try to kill the snake: at best this wastes time; at worst it may lead to another victim.
- Don't give the victim alcoholic beverages or coffee.
- Apply a constricting band. If there's going to be a long delay—4 or 5 hours, for example—before the victim receives emergency care, and if the bite was to an arm, hand, or leg, you should apply a constricting band about 2 to 4 inches above the bite.

A constricting band is a strip of cloth about ¾ to ½ inch wide tied around a limb but kept loose enough to insert a finger underneath it. Loosen the band if it becomes too tight, but don't remove it. The object of constricting bands is to slow the movement of snake venom away from the bite.

Scorpions

Scorpions look like little crabs. The segmented tail curls over the body and ends with a stinger. Most species are about 3 inches long; they're black or yellowish in color. Scorpions are common throughout the southwest; the two most dangerous species live in Arizona.

Scorpions don't attack humans, but they often get

Scorpion venom

In equal measures, scorpion venom is more poisonous than snake venom. However, scorpions inject a smaller amount of venom.

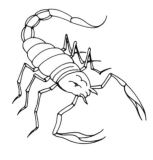

Gila monster

The gila monster and the related Mexican beaded lizard are the world's only poisonous lizards. The Mexican beaded lizard can be found only in Mexico; the gila monster lives in the deserts of the southwest, particularly in Arizona, southern Utah, and New Mexico.

into shoes or clothing or are stepped on at night. The stings of most scorpions are comparatively harmless; the venom of the dangerous species (found in Arizona) contains a neurotoxin and is potentially lethal.

The immediate symptom of a scorpion sting is a severe, sharp, burning pain. **If the sting was of a nonlethal scorpion,** the area of the sting will become swollen and discolored. **If the sting was of a lethal scorpion,** the sharp pain produced by the sting is quickly followed by a pins-and-needles sensation at the sting area. The area of the sting will not become swollen and will not become discolored; within 1 to 3 hours the following symptoms will appear: itching of eyes, nose, and throat; tightness of jaw muscles and difficulty speaking; extreme restlessness and muscle twitching; muscle spasms with pain, nausea, vomiting, and incontinence; drowsiness; and difficulty breathing and irregular pulse.

In the event of a scorpion sting:
• Contact medical help immediately, whether or not you believe the sting to have been of a lethal scorpion.
• Keep the victim calm.
• Apply ice packs to the sting.
• Apply a constricting band as near the site of the sting as possible. Locate the band between the sting and the victim's heart.

Poisonous spiders

The United States is home to two species of poisonous spider: the black widow and the brown recluse. The females of both species are more deadly than the males.

Black widow

The black widow has a globe-shaped, shiny black body about ½ inch long and a leg span of about 2 inches. There's a red or orange hourglass-shaped mark on the belly; on some spiders this is replaced by several triangles or spots.

Black widow spiders build their webs under or between rocks, under loose bark, around outdoor water faucets, and in woodpiles, garages, basements, and sheds.

Follow these routine precautions to avoid encounters with black widow spiders:
• Hose under steps and around windows and doors. If an area becomes infested, spray with an insecticide.
• Wear gloves and a long-sleeved shirt when working

Spiders in outhouses
In bygone days, encounters with black widow spiders were common in outhouses; the seats offered the spiders ideal web locations. Look before you sit.

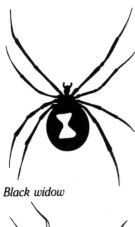

Black widow

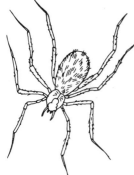

Brown recluse

Tarantulas
Tarantulas may not be pleasant to look at, but they aren't poisonous. A tarantula bite usually feels like a pinprick, and there may be swelling around the wound—but that's about all.

in spider-infested areas, such as around woodpiles or in sheds.

The bite of a black widow spider usually feels like a sharp, stinging pinprick, but some bites go unnoticed. There may be slight swelling and two tiny puncture marks at the site of the bite. The bite is followed by dull, numbing pain, which usually increases in intensity, reaching its peak in 1 to 3 hours; it may continue for 12 to 48 hours.

Within 10 to 40 minutes of the bite, the venom, which attacks the nerves, causes abdominal muscles to become rigid—they may feel boardlike. This is accompanied by stomach pain and muscle spasms in the extremities. Both of these symptoms usually subside within 48 hours. The victim may have difficulty breathing and swallowing. Other symptoms include convulsions, paralysis, delirium, nausea, vomiting, sweating, drooping eyelids, headache, and fever.

In the event of a black widow (or other) spider bite, call a doctor immediately. Keep the victim warm and calm.

Brown recluse, or violin, spider

The brown recluse has a brown or fawn-colored body about ½ inch long and a leg span of about 2 inches. It has a dark, violin-shaped mark on its back.

Although sometimes found outdoors, most brown recluse spiders are house spiders: they spin their webs in dark, undisturbed areas inside homes or outbuildings such as woodsheds. They're called "recluse" because they frequently hide in closets, dresser drawers, the folds of clothing or bedding, garages, attics, or sheds. They aren't aggressive and will try to escape when threatened. Most bites are the result of trapping the spider, for example, when the victim puts on clothing in which the spider is hiding or steps on a wandering spider at night.

Follow these precautions to avoid encounters with brown recluse spiders:
• Shake out clothing and bedding before use.
• Clean beneath and behind furniture.
• Remove spiders, webs, and egg cases from living and storage areas.

The bite of a brown recluse causes very little if any pain. Within 2 to 8 hours the pain will become severe, and the area of the bite will become red. Brown recluse venom contains a substance destructive to tissue that causes a large spreading sore. A blister will

What happens with an insect sting

When you're stung by a bee or other insect, your body's immune system responds by releasing antibodies, substances that counteract the harmful effects of germs and toxins. Our bodies produce specific antibodies in response to specific germs and toxins. Some people, though, over-react and release too much antibody, which becomes life-threatening. Allergic reactions to bee stings are more common in adults than in children simply because adults have had the time to gradually develop a serious allergy to the venom. Any bad reaction to a sting should be considered a forewarning of more violent reactions to come.

Dangerous stings

The severity of a bee sting frequently depends on its location. If a bee is swallowed or inhaled, it may sting the inside of the throat, and the swelling can cause strangulation. A sting to the neck can also affect breathing. Because bee stingers don't disintegrate and can't be absorbed by the body, a sting to the area of the eye can be dangerous: even after months or years, the stinger can scratch the eye. A stinger embedded in an eyelid must be removed surgically.

form at the wound, becoming dark and hard within 3 to 4 days. This sore will become star-shaped and deep purple; within 2 weeks it will have formed an open ulcer.

The bite can cause further general reactions, particularly in children. These may include fever, chills, weakness, nausea, vomiting, joint pain, an all-over "sick" feeling, and possibly a generalized rash or small reddish or purplish spots.

In the event of a brown recluse (or other) spider bite, call a doctor immediately.

Bees and wasps

For most of us, a bee sting is only a minor annoyance: a sharp pinprick followed by several minutes of pain. The area of the sting becomes red and swollen, and it itches and burns for a few hours. It's an unpleasant experience, but it doesn't last long. That's the normal reaction to a bee sting.

For some people, however, a bee sting presents serious danger. An estimated 1 to 2 million Americans are severely allergic to the venom of bees, wasps, hornets, and yellow jackets. When stung, they suffer soreness and swelling not only at the site of the sting but also on other parts of the body. They can experience fever, chills, and light-headedness; hives, joint and muscle pains, and swelling of the lymph glands may also occur. Other severe reactions may include a sudden drop in blood pressure with loss of consciousness, difficulty breathing, shock, and—for about 50 to 100 people each year—death.

If you've ever had a bad reaction to a bee sting, you're probably allergic and should carry an emergency self-treatment kit. These are available only with a doctor's prescription. Each kit contains antihistamine tablets, alcohol swabs, and a preloaded syringe filled with the drug adrenaline, which works extremely well in counteracting the allergic response. If you give yourself an injection as soon as symptoms appear, you can avoid a dangerous reaction.

The best way to prevent painful encounters with stinging insects is to stay away from them.

Hornets and wasps don't usually attack unless their nest is threatened. Yellow jackets, however, are very aggressive and quick-tempered. Many reported "bee" stings turn out to be yellow jacket stings.

To prevent insect stings:

• Avoid outdoor activities near stinging insects. Ho-

Telling bees apart

Honeybees have round, smooth abdomens; bumblebees, which are two to three times larger than honeybees, have round, furry abdomens. Hornets, yellow jackets, and other wasps have long, slender abdomens. The bodies of all these insects are usually striped yellow and black. Bumblebees are large and make a noisy buzzing.

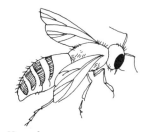

Honeybee

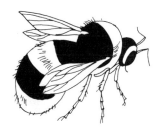

Bumblebee

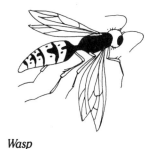

Wasp

neybees and bumblebees can be found around flowers; wasps and yellow jackets in orchards or around garbage; hornets in the woods. Stay away from garbage cans and hollow trees.
• Don't wear fragrant cosmetics, perfumes, or hair spray when outdoors during insect season.
• Don't wear bright-colored clothes. Don't wear red or black—both attract bees. Flowery prints are also a bad idea. Instead, wear light colors, such as white, green, tan, and khaki. Long sleeves and long pants are best; loose-fitting clothes should be avoided because stinging insects can become trapped in them.
• Don't go barefoot. Wear closed shoes or sneakers; most sandals don't offer much protection.
• Keep food covered outdoors, especially sweet foods and drinks.
• Move slowly or stand still in the vicinity of bees. Most stings can be easily handled.
• Remove the stinger. Don't use tweezers to remove a bee's stinger. Squeezing the stinger will release more venom into the wound. Scrape away the stinger with a fingernail or the edge of a knife blade.
• Wash the wound with soap and water and apply an antiseptic.
• If available, apply ice to the wound. This will help reduce the swelling.
• The pain and irritation can be relieved by applying a paste made from baking soda and water; some doctors recommend applying meat tenderizer (any brand will do). Make a paste of ¼ tsp meat tenderizer added to about 1 or 2 tsp water. Rubbed into the wound, this will quickly stop the pain.

Ticks

Ticks are common in woods and fields throughout the United States. They have flat, brown, speckled bodies about ¼ inch long and eight legs. These tiny insects are bloodsucking parasites: they attach themselves to a suitable host—frequently a human—by biting and burrowing their heads into the host's skin. They reinforce the attachment with a cementlike secretion; some ticks also inject a neurotoxin that serves as a digestive aid.

Prevention of tick bites

Ticks are found most frequently in warm weather in wooded areas. They're common in tall grasses—they climb to the top of the grass and wait for a suitable

Rocky Mountain spotted fever and Lyme disease

Ticks are known to transmit several diseases, including Rocky Mountain spotted fever and Lyme disease.

Rocky Mountain spotted fever isn't confined to the Rocky Mountains—cases have been diagnosed as far east as Long Island. It's caused by a bacteria-like organism called rickettsia that the tick deposits in the victim while sucking blood. The symptoms of the disease begin about 7 days after a tick bite and include fever, chills, muscle pain, and a severe headache. About 4 days later, a rose-colored rash usually appears on the wrists, ankles, and forearms. The treatment for Rocky Mountain spotted fever is antibiotics.

Lyme disease was first recognized in 1976; it's named for the Connecticut town where it was discovered (it has now been reported in more than 15 other states). The first symptom of Lyme disease, a circular rash at the site of the bite, usually appears about a week after the bite. As the rash spreads outward, its center clears. Similar lesions may appear, usually clearing up in a few weeks. Other symptoms include swollen glands, sore throat, tiredness (fatigue), extreme weakness, fever, vomiting, muscle pains, and joint pain. These usually go away on their own. However, arthritic symptoms may start about a month after the rash and can recur over a period of years. These symptoms usually affect the victim's knees.

The treatment for Lyme disease is antibiotics. If begun soon enough after the infection, this treatment can prevent more serious symptoms, but even without treatment, the disease doesn't seem to be fatal.

victim to pass by. Follow these precautions in tick-infested areas:

• Wear long sleeves, long pants, and high-topped shoes or boots. Tight cuffs at the ankles and wrists help; tuck your pants into your shoes or boots. A tight-fitting cap is also a good idea—ticks are sometimes contacted on tree branches and leaves.
• Use repellents. Cover exposed skin, such as ankles, lower legs, wrists, and arms with the repellent. Clothing can be dipped in or sprayed with the repellent.
• Inspect your body thoroughly once or twice daily. Pay special attention to your armpits, neck, ears, crotch, and groin. Look for anything unfamiliar; when engorged with blood, ticks are no longer brown but can be grayish and oval in shape.
• Brush clothing, hang it up outdoors, and leave it there several hours. Brushing clothes may not remove all ticks; ticks still on your clothes after brushing will leave after several hours.

If you find a tick anywhere on your body, you must remove it. If the tick isn't yet embedded, you can brush it off. Don't try to yank or twist out ticks that have dug in, since any squeezing may inject more toxin into the wound, and you may yank off part of the tick but leave its head still embedded in your skin.

Cover the tick with a tissue or gauze pad saturated with alcohol or mineral oil. This will block the tick's

Where to look for ticks

Ticks usually crawl upward on victims, but they stop at constricting clothing. Check around the waist, bra line, top of socks, and similar spots. Don't forget to check your scalp and ears.

Pets that have been in the woods should be inspected daily.

Ticks don't immediately begin to feed on their human hosts, so frequent inspections of your body and prompt removal of any ticks can diminish the risk of tick bites and the diseases caused by tick bites.

breathing pores and cause it to withdraw. You can achieve the same result by coating the tick with Vaseline, fingernail polish, mineral oil, salad oil, or machine oil. If the tick still holds on, put a heated needle, lighted cigarette, or match close to but not on the tick; the heat may make it release its grip. The tick can then be removed with tweezers. Immediately after removing the tick, wash the area and your hands thoroughly with soap and water.

If you become ill with fever, headache, and rash, contact a doctor. Inform the doctor of any tick bite.

Poisonous fish

Several kinds of fish are capable of inflicting painful, poisonous stings. Those most frequently encountered include stingrays, catfish, weever fish, scorpion fish, toadfish, stargazers, surgeonfish, and sea urchins. In most cases, the poison is injected through spines. Although deaths from these fish are rare, their stings can be exceedingly painful.

• Handle any unfamiliar fish with caution and use extreme caution—or avoid—handling any fish with spines.

• Wear shoes or foot protection when walking through water in search of shells or when fishing; shuffle your feet.

• Don't stick your hands in underwater rock crevices.

• Be careful when removing fish from hooks or nets. If you have any doubts about a fish, cut the line and let the fish go.

The stings of these fish cause immediate stinging or throbbing pain. The pain may stay at the site of the wound or may spread throughout the body and last for several hours or even days. The pain from some fish stings is so intense that victims have been known to lose consciousness. There may be redness and swelling at the site of the sting, and the area may become numb.

Other symptoms depend on the species of fish and may include vomiting, diarrhea, fainting, sweating, muscle cramps, irregular pulse, possible paralysis, difficulty breathing, and convulsions.

In the event of a fish sting, contact medical help immediately. Flush the wound with fresh or salt water. After flushing the wound, soak the affected area in hot water or put hot compresses on it. The water should be as hot as the victim can tolerate (122° F. is recommended); the heat will deactivate the poison.

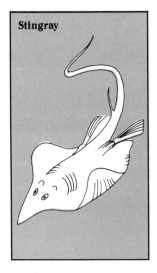

Stingray

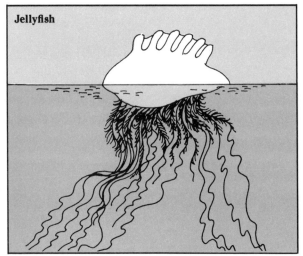

Jellyfish

Don't panic
One of the greatest dangers of stings from poisonous fish and jellyfish is panic: the sting may not cause much harm, but the victim many panic and drown.

Continue the application of hot water for 30 minutes to 1 hour.

Jellyfish

Jellyfish, Portuguese men-of-war, corals, and sea anemones have tentacles that can penetrate human skin and inject venom. Jellyfish and Portuguese men-of-war float on the surface of the water, trailing tentacles; sea anemones and corals form colonies or attach themselves to submerged objects. These creatures, most common in tropical waters, pose hazards for swimmers and divers.

Stings from tentacles cause severe burning pain; a red, weltlike sore forms at the site of the wound. Some victims (depending on the species of fish) experience headache, nausea, vomiting, muscle cramps, diarrhea, convulsions, and breathing difficulties.

In the event of a sting from one of these fish, contact medical help immediately.

Alcohol poured over the wound will deactivate the venom. Calamine lotion spread over the area will help relieve the burning. Tentacles may cling to the victim's skin. Remove them gently with a towel; don't try to remove them with your hands.

11

Food Poisoning

Ptomaine poisoning
"Ptomaine" poisoning isn't the same as food poisoning. Ptomaines are substances produced by decaying animal or vegetable proteins. Foods containing ptomaines usually look spoiled, smell awful, and taste worse. For these reasons, people rarely eat them. What's more, most ptomaines aren't harmful. Most so-called ptomaine poisonings are actually staphylococcal poisonings.

Eggs and their protective shells
Uncooked eggs with intact shells are well protected from contamination; once they're cooked, however, eggs are no longer protected. Bacteria can pass right through the unbroken shells of cooked eggs.

Children love Easter egg hunts, and they usually find the eggs in less time than it took to hide them. Such was the case at one particular Easter egg hunt in California a few years ago. More than 3,500 eggs had been hidden; 300 gleeful children charged out to find them. Within 20 minutes, all the colored eggs had been scooped up, and the children were happily peeling and eating them.

A few hours later, many of these children were no longer happy: they were suffering vomiting, diarrhea, and stomach cramps—sure signs of food poisoning.

Poisoned by Easter eggs? Medical researchers quickly identified this tale's villain: the cook. He had spent quite a while preparing the 3,500 eggs, cooking them, cooling them in cold water, and then dying them. When he'd finished, he found he didn't have room to refrigerate all the eggs, so he stored them at room temperature for the three days before the hunt.

What the cook didn't know was that he was carrying the disease-causing bacteria *Staphylococcus* in his nose and throat. At some point during the preparation of the eggs, he had transmitted bacteria onto the eggs or into the water in which they were cooling. Perhaps he sneezed, or perhaps he just forgot to wash his hands before handling the eggs. At room temperature for so many days, the bacteria had an ideal environment in which to multiply.

Food poisoning usually results from poor food-handling practices, usually strikes more than one person, and is usually mild. More important, it can usually be prevented. Had the cook washed his hands and avoided sneezing around the eggs, he wouldn't have spread the germs. Or had he promptly put the eggs into a refrigerator when they were done, the bacteria wouldn't have multiplied.

The sources of food poisoning

Most kinds of food poisoning are caused by bacteria. Bacteria are everywhere—in water, in soil, inside us, and inside the food we prepare or eat. They're not all harmful, but some, such as the *Staphylococcus* bacteria carried by the cook, cause illness. Bacteria can cause food poisoning in two ways. First, disease-

Food, warmth, and moisture

To grow and multiply, bacteria need food, warmth, and moisture. Most bacteria can survive in frozen food, and bacteria can be transferred from one food to another on utensils or hands. At room temperature, bacteria in food multiply and may produce toxins. This is why outbreaks of food poisoning are common during summer months, when perishable foods are carried to picnics and cookouts.

producing bacteria can enter our bodies in contaminated food. Second, given a chance, bacteria in food can produce toxins. Eating the food—and the toxins—causes illness.

Several different kinds of bacteria contaminate the foods we eat. Some of these bacteria regularly appear in certain foods. *Salmonella* bacteria, for example, are frequently found in raw poultry and meat. Some bacteria can get into foods from the people who handle them. *Staphylococcus* bacteria are commonly carried by people on their hands, in droplets from their nose and throat, or in pus from sores. When these bacteria come in contact with certain foods, they multiply if the conditions are right. *Staphylococcus* bacteria won't multiply on raw vegetables or fruit, but they'll rapidly multiply in cream-filled pastries (or Easter eggs) at the right temperature. Cooking and refrigeration control the growth of bacteria in foods, but often foods become contaminated and cause illness simply because they aren't handled properly.

Food poisoning can also be caused by viruses, protozoa, and molds. Viruses and protozoa are present in the human intestinal tract and can get into food when a person fails to wash his or her hands after a visit to the bathroom and then handles food. Molds grow on improperly stored food.

Prevention of food poisoning

You can protect yourself and others by being aware of the variety of ways in which foods can become contaminated. The most common causes of food poisoning are lack of sanitation in the handling of food, improper storage of food, and improper preparation and cooking of food.

1. Sanitary handling of food. Sanitary handling of food helps prevent most food poisoning. Make sure your hands, hair, fingernails, and clothing are clean before working with food, and wash your hands whenever your work is interrupted.

A bug that's going around

An estimated 2 million cases of food poisoning occur in the United States each year. Many cases of food poisoning go unreported, however, because people frequently attribute an "upset stomach" caused by food poisoning to "a bug that's going around."

• Wash your hands before and after handling raw foods.

• Wash your hands after using the toilet or changing a baby's diaper.

• Wash your hands after smoking, blowing your nose, or petting the dog (what's your dog doing in the kitchen?).

• Avoid using your hands to mix foods: clean utensils are a much better idea.

Keeping wooden tools clean

Wash wooden utensils and cutting boards periodically in a solution of 2 parts water and 1 part bleach. Rinse thoroughly.

Saving time

If you cook foods ahead of time, put them in the refrigerator until you're ready to serve them. This includes eggs, which should be promptly refrigerated and kept chilled until you're ready to use them.

Salmonella *in poultry*

Salmonella *bacteria are often present in poultry, even when it's frozen. When you cut up a chicken, the bacteria get on the knife; if you then use the knife to cut something else, you contaminate this second food with the* Salmonella *bacteria. Avoid this so-called cross-contamination by washing knives after each use.*

• Keep your hands away from your mouth, nose, and hair.
• Cover coughs and sneezes with tissues—and wash your hands.
• Wear plastic gloves if you have a cut or an infection on your hands.
• Wash dust or dirt off the tops of cans before opening them.
• Handle dishes by the edges, glasses by the base, and silverware by the handles.
• Scrape dishes before washing them, and wash them in hot, soapy water.
• Keep all dishes, utensils, kitchen equipment, and work surfaces clean.
• Wash cutting boards, work surfaces, and utensils with hot, soapy water before and after use with raw poultry or meat. Wash them thoroughly before you use them with anything else, raw or cooked.
• Wash knives between uses, particularly if the knife is used on raw poultry or meat.
• Don't allow your pet's dishes, toys, or bedding in the kitchen or near anything that may come in contact with food, utensils, or working surfaces used in food preparation.
2. Proper storage of food. Keeping foods cold prevents the growth of bacteria. Refrigeration doesn't kill bacteria but keeps them from multiplying and retards the ability of some bacteria to produce toxins. From the moment you buy food, you're responsible for its care—safe use of foods begins in the grocery store.
• Make the grocery store your last stop, and take your food home immediately.
• Select meats near the end of shopping, and select frozen foods and dairy products last.
• Don't buy food in cracked or torn packages, and don't buy partially defrosted frozen foods.
• Make certain that your frozen food purchases are put in plastic bags.
• Buy perishable foods in small quantities so you won't keep them too long.
• Put foods in your refrigerator as soon as you get them home.
• Store poultry and meat in the plastic wrapping they come in for only a day or two; for longer storage, remove the store wrapping and wrap loosely in wax paper or plastic wrap. If you're going to freeze these products, wrap them tightly and date them—use older items first. *(text continued on page 84)*

Food poisoning

This chart lists the major types of food poisoning, the foods most often involved, and the symptoms caused by each. As you'll notice, the symptoms of most food poisonings are mild. Some are so mild that the poisoning is barely noticed or is passed off as an upset stomach. Some, however, can be dangerous to children, the elderly, or the infirm; and botulism can be deadly to anyone.

Type of poisoning	Sources	Symptoms
Salmonellosis; caused by *Salmonella* bacteria	Raw meats, poultry, eggs, fish, milk, and foods made with them. (Marijuana and small pet turtles are both prime sources of *Salmonella* bacteria.) Bacteria multiply rapidly at room temperature.	Onset: 12 to 48 hours after eating (or smoking marijuana or handling a pet turtle). Severe headache, nausea, fever, stomach cramps, diarrhea; sometimes vomiting. Usually lasts 2 to 7 days and can be fatal in infants, the elderly, and the infirm.
Staphylococcal, "staph," food poisoning; caused by *Staphylococcus aureus* bacteria	Can develop in any food left too long at room temperature. Chief sources are tuna, egg, chicken, potato, and macaroni salads; egg products, custards, cream-filled pastries; meats, including ham and salami, and poultry.	Onset: 1 to 8 hours after eating. Diarrhea, vomiting, nausea, abdominal cramps, exhaustion. Lasts 24 to 48 hours. Usually mild, it's often attributed to other causes, such as the flu.
Perfringens food poisoning; caused by *Clostridium perfringens* bacteria	Meat, poultry, and foods made with them, including stews, soups, and gravies. Bacteria multiply rapidly at room temperature and are destroyed by cooking.	Onset: 8 to 22 hours after eating. Stomach pain and diarrhea; sometimes nausea and vomiting. Lasts about 24 to 48 hours and is usually mild but can be serious in the elderly or infirm.
Botulism; caused by *Clostridium botulinum* bacteria	These bacteria are everywhere but produce toxin only in an anaerobic (oxygen-less) environment of low acidity. Improperly canned low-acid foods (especially home-canned) such as green beans, corn, beets, peppers, mushrooms, spinach, olives, beef are chief sources.	Onset: 8 hours to 8 days after eating. Symptoms usually begin with nausea, vomiting, diarrhea, and stomach cramps; then weakness, blurred or double vision, headache, difficulty swallowing, slurred speech, drooping eyelids, dilated pupils, and progressive paralysis, including the respiratory muscles. Usually lasts 3 to 6 days but can be fatal. Get help immediately.
Shigellosis (bacillary dysentery); caused by *Shigella* bacteria	Milk and dairy products, poultry, mixed salads (fish, poultry, potato, macaroni, and egg). Can develop in any moist food that is not thoroughly cooked; bacteria multiply rapidly at or above room temperature.	Onset: 1 to 7 days after eating. Stomach pain, cramps, diarrhea, fever; sometimes vomiting, with blood or mucus in stool. Can be serious in infants, the elderly, and the infirm.
Campylobacterosis; caused by *Campylobacter jejuni* bacteria	Raw poultry, meat, and unpasteurized milk.	Onset: 2 to 5 days after eating. Diarrhea, stomach cramps, fever; sometimes bloody stool. Lasts 2 to 7 days.

Type of poisoning	Sources	Symptoms
Bacterial gastroenteritis; caused by *Yersinia enterocolitica* bacteria	Meat, water, raw vegetables, and unpasteurized milk. Bacteria multiply rapidly at room temperature.	Onset: 2 to 5 days after eating. Fever, headache, nausea, diarrhea, sick feeling; often mistaken for the flu. Common in children but can affect people of all ages.
Cereus food poisoning; caused by *Bacillus cereus* bacteria	Raw foods. Bacteria multiply rapidly at room temperature.	Onset: 1 to 18 hours after eating. May cause stomach pain and diarrhea or nausea and vomiting. Rarely lasts longer than 1 day.
Cholera; caused by *Vibrio cholera* bacteria	Fish and shellfish harvested from waters contaminated by human sewage. Chief sources are fish and shellfish eaten raw, such as oysters.	Onset: 1 to 3 days after eating. Symptoms can range from mild diarrhea to life-threatening dehydration from intense diarrhea. Severe cases require hospitalization.
Parahaemolyticus food poisoning; caused by *Vibrio parahaemolyticus* bacteria	Fish and shellfish; caused by bacteria that live in salt water and thrive in warm weather.	Onset: 15 to 24 hours after eating. Nausea, vomiting, stomach cramps, diarrhea; sometimes fever, headache, chills, mucus or blood in the stool. Lasts 1 to 2 days and is rarely fatal.
Viral gastroenteritis; caused by various viruses	Found in human intestinal tract and feces. Can be introduced to food when sewage is used as fertilizer; when food handlers don't wash hands; when shellfish are harvested from waters contaminated by sewage.	Onset: after 24 hours. Diarrhea, nausea, vomiting, breathing difficulties. Usually lasts 4 to 5 days but may go on for weeks.
Hepatitis A; caused by hepatitis A virus, which is different from the infectious variety (hepatitis B)	Shellfish harvested from contaminated waters and foods, such as vegetables, that are handled a lot during preparation and then eaten raw.	Onset: 2 to 6 weeks. Fever, weakness, loss of appetite, jaundice (yellowing of skin and whites of eyes). Severe cases cause liver damage and may be fatal.
Mycotoxicosis; caused by mold toxins	Toxins are produced in foods that are high in moisture, such as beans and grains, stored in a moist place.	May cause liver or kidney damage.
Giardiasis; caused by *Giardia lamblia* protozoa	Found in the human intestinal tract and feces. Can be introduced to food when sewage is used as fertilizer or when food handlers don't wash hands. Chief sources are foods that are handled a lot during preparation.	Diarrhea, stomach pains, gas, loss of appetite, nausea, vomiting.
Amebiasis (amoebic dysentery); caused by *Entamoeba histolytica* (amebic protozoa)	Found in the human intestinal tract and feces. Can be introduced to food when sewage is used as fertilizer or when food handlers don't wash hands. Chief sources are foods that are handled a lot during preparation.	Tenderness over the colon or liver, loose morning stools, recurrent diarrhea, nervousness, weight loss, and fatigue. The blood disorder anemia may develop.

• Check stored food periodically and throw away any food that has grown moldy, shriveled, and discolored or has a strange odor.

3. Preparing and cooking food.

• Don't thaw food at room temperature. Either thaw foods in the refrigerator or begin cooking them before they're thawed. If you're really in a hurry, submerge them in warm water.

• Clean poultry thoroughly. Cooking isn't the sole precaution necessary for the prevention of salmonellosis. Poultry should always be rinsed carefully. Remember that any utensils or work surfaces used in the preparation of raw poultry must be thoroughly cleaned before being used again.

• Never allow raw meats or poultry to touch foods that are eaten raw.

• Heat foods thoroughly. Cooking foods at high temperatures kills bacteria. High heat is especially important when preparing such foods as milk, milk products, eggs, meat, poultry, fish, and shellfish.

When cooking meats and poultry, use a meat thermometer to make sure the interior cooks thoroughly. Insert the thermometer in the center of the thickest portion of the meat or poultry. Poultry and pork should reach an internal temperature of 165° F.; beef should reach at least 140° F.

• Serve hot foods hot and cold foods cold. Time the cooking of hot foods so that they can be served while they're still hot; if there's going to be a delay, keep the temperature of hot foods at or above 140° F. Serve cold food directly from the refrigerator. Bacteria grow rapidly at temperatures between 60° and 125° F. (see chart, page 88).

• Stuff poultry immediately before roasting. Don't jam the stuffing into the bird; put it in lightly to allow heat to penetrate. Make sure the stuffing reaches a temperature of at least 165° F. during cooking.

• Don't leave leftover foods on the table, but store them in the refrigerator promptly. Put both hot and cold foods in the refrigerator. You don't need to wait for hot foods to cool off before refrigerating them; put them in shallow dishes so they'll cool quickly inside the refrigerator.

• Reheat leftovers thoroughly. Leftovers should be reheated to at least 165° F.; gravies should be heated until they reach a rolling boil.

• Avoid raw fish, raw meats, and raw (unpasteurized) milk. Many people decide to avoid the potential dangers of these foods by avoiding them altogether.

Handling stuffing
Don't stuff uncooked meat, poultry, or fish and then put it in the refrigerator. If you make stuffing in advance, store it separately. Remove any stuffing before refrigerating leftover meat, poultry, or fish; store the stuffing in a separate container—do the same with any broth or gravy.

Is your refrigerator cold enough?
Make sure your refrigerator temperature is cold enough to keep foods safe. If foods are to be kept for only 3 or 4 days, the temperature should be 45° F.; if foods are to be kept longer, the temperature should be 40° F. or lower.

Trichinosis

Trichinella spiralis, *a tiny worm frequently found in the muscles of pork, causes a disease known as trichinosis. To prevent trichinosis, all pork or pork products must be cooked thoroughly (to at least 170° F.). If you can't use a thermometer, be certain the pork is cooked until there's no trace of pink in the meat or juices.*

Food poisoning and diarrhea

Diarrhea that results from food poisoning is an example of your body's ability to protect itself. Instead of allowing harmful bacteria or viruses to get into the system through the walls of the intestinal tract, your body speeds up its elimination process, producing frequent loose or watery stools. Diarrhea usually ends within 18 hours without the aid of antidiarrhea medicine. Indeed, by taking or giving such medicines in the case of food poisoning, you might only interfere with the self-purging process.

Clostridium botulinum *spores and honey*

Although not dangerous to most people, C. botulinum *spores can make infants sick. Since honey of any type can contain* C. botulinum *spores, you shouldn't feed honey to children under 1 year old.*

Botulism

Botulism is the most serious type of food poisoning. Although very rare, it's very deadly: approximately two-thirds of the people who suffer botulism poisoning die, and recovery is slow for those who survive.

Clostridium botulinum bacteria are everywhere: in the air and water and in the foods we eat. When they're in the spore, or inactive, state, they're harmless to most people. The bacteria remain inactive and harmless unless they're put into an anaerobic (oxygen-less) environment. If certain other conditions are right, they then begin to grow and produce one of the most lethal toxins known—it's 7 million times more potent than cobra venom. This toxin causes botulism.

Where can you find an anaerobic environment? Inside a sealed can or jar. Incidents of botulism poisoning from commercially canned foods are very rare, for commercial canners follow strict safety rules, and they're checked continuously by the Food and Drug Administration (FDA). Therefore, most cases of botulism poisoning involve home-preserved foods.

Home-canned foods are usually hermetically sealed or made airtight in their containers. This helps prevent spoilage, but it also presents any *C. botulinum* spores in the food with the perfect anaerobic environment. However, the absence of oxygen is only one of the conditions necessary for the growth of the toxin. The spores won't grow in foods that have high acid, sugar, or salt content. Canned fruit juices, jams and jellies, sauerkraut, most tomato products, and heavily salted hams are foods in which the spores won't grow; green beans, corn, beets, peppers, and meat are examples of foods in which the spores can grow.

In addition to these conditions, the home-canned foods must be at a suitable temperature. The ideal temperature is 78° to 96° F., but the spores can survive being boiled.

Heating home-canned food well beyond the boiling point will kill *C. botulinum* spores. This can be done in a pressure cooker, following guidelines established by the U.S. Department of Agriculture. *C. botulinum* spores can't be destroyed by freezing.

Avoiding botulism

Both home-canned foods and, rarely, commercially canned foods can contain botulism. How can you

If you home can foods

If you home can foods, follow the instructions provided in U.S. Department of Agriculture publications. These publications are available (you'll have to pay for them) from the Superintendent of Documents, Government Printing Office, Washington, D.C. 20402. These are only a few of the available publications; write for a list:

Home Canning of Fruits and Vegetables (HG-8)

Home Canning of Meat and Poultry (HG-106)

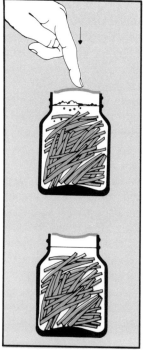

Safety test
Before you open home-canned food, check the lid with a fingertip. If the lid bulges, discard the food; don't taste even a drop of it. If the lid is depressed and doesn't yield under your fingertips, then the seal is safe.

avoid it?

When the *C. botulinum* spores grow, they give off gas, and the gas can make cans and jars lose their vacuum seal. Jars sometimes burst; cans swell. Avoid food containers with leaky seals and bent or bulging cans. If you open a can and find the food spoiled or if its color or odor don't seem right, don't taste the food—don't even sniff it closely. Botulism can be deadly even in tiny amounts. If it's home-canned, throw it away where no person or animal can get to it. If it's commercially canned, call the store where you bought it, your county health department, or the nearest FDA office.

Treatment for food poisoning

If more than one person gets sick a few hours after a shared meal, you can be pretty sure it's food poisoning. You may even know the cause—thinking back, everyone may agree that the tuna salad did taste a little odd—but there's really no way you can determine which food poisoning you're suffering from. See your doctor if you're more than mildly ill. For some food poisonings, prescription medicines are necessary; for most, no treatment other than rest is needed.

The greatest danger of most food poisonings is loss of fluid. Vomiting and diarrhea are your body's natural response to toxins—your body is trying to rid itself of the poison. Along with the poison, however, your body will get rid of necessary fluids, and you may become dehydrated—dried out. If this dehydration is serious, you may need to be hospitalized and given fluids intravenously.

Botulism is an exception. Unlike other food poisonings, botulism only sometimes involves vomiting and diarrhea; instead, the toxin affects the nervous system. Botulism is a life-threatening disease—see a doctor immediately if you have any reason to suspect botulism. There is an antitoxin to the *C. botulinum* toxin, and hospitalization is required.

Shellfish poisoning

The shellfish we eat aren't poisonous, but they can become contaminated when the water they live in is contaminated. Certain kinds of shellfish—oysters, clams, and mussels—are particularly prone to contamination because of the way they take food and oxygen from the water around them. They pump water across their gills, filtering out the substances, such as the tiny organisms called plankton, that form their

Red tide
The organisms that cause red tide are closely moni- tored: warning signs are posted when concentrations reach dangerous levels.

diet. In this way, they also take into their bodies any bacteria, viruses, or other contaminants that happen to be in the water. They do such a good job of filtering that the level of harmful bacteria in a shellfish can be up to 20 times that of the water around it.

Sometimes the plankton shellfish eat are poisonous. During the warmer months, a species of plankton known as *Gonyaulax catanella* appears in certain areas. These tiny organisms rapidly multiply until they color the ocean waters for many miles. Because the color is usually pink or red, the appearance of these organisms has come to be known as "red tide."

These plankton produce a poison, known as sax- itoxin, that causes paralytic shellfish poisoning (PSP). This poison blocks nerve impulses, causing paralysis of the respiratory muscles. It's so deadly that eating one contaminated shellfish could kill a person.

The shellfish industry works closely with state health agencies and the FDA to ensure that the shell- fish we eat come from safe waters. State agencies prohibit shellfish harvesting in areas contaminated by sewage, industrial wastes, or the organisms that cause PSP. Thanks to their efforts, typhoid fever and cholera are today rarely transmitted by shellfish.

Prevention of shellfish poisoning

The following precautions will help you avoid food poisoning from shellfish:

• Don't buy shellfish from roadside stands. Most cases of illness caused by shellfish consumption can be traced to illegally harvested shellfish. Don't take chances: buy your shellfish in a grocery store or fish market.

• Keep all seafood refrigerated at between 32° and 40° F.

• Don't store seafood for long periods. Even kept cold, seafood will deteroriate, allowing bacteria to multiply.

• Wash your hands before and after handling seafood.

• Cook shellfish thoroughly. Most instances of shell- fish poisoning are the result of eating shellfish raw. Many people choose to avoid all raw fish (along with raw meats and raw—unpasteurized—milk).

Cooking will kill bacteria, but only very high heat will destroy the hepatitis A virus. No amount of clean- ing or cooking will destroy the toxins that cause PSP.

• Eat shellfish only in months that have an "r" in their name. This old adage has a lot of merit. Months that

Warning
People with liver disease shouldn't eat raw seafood of any kind. One species of bacteria found in seafood has been shown to cause fever, chills, and prostra- tion in people with liver disease.

don't have an "r" in their name are the warmer months, the months during which the organisms that cause PSP usually appear. Furthermore, shellfish eat less and therefore accumulate fewer harmful bacteria in their bodies during cold weather.

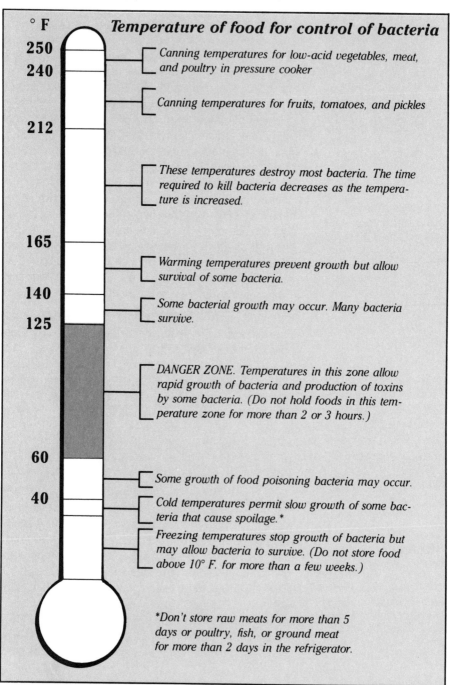

Temperature of food for control of bacteria

°F

250
240 — Canning temperatures for low-acid vegetables, meat, and poultry in pressure cooker

— Canning temperatures for fruits, tomatoes, and pickles

212

— These temperatures destroy most bacteria. The time required to kill bacteria decreases as the temperature is increased.

165 — Warming temperatures prevent growth but allow survival of some bacteria.

140 — Some bacterial growth may occur. Many bacteria survive.

125

— DANGER ZONE. Temperatures in this zone allow rapid growth of bacteria and production of toxins by some bacteria. (Do not hold foods in this temperature zone for more than 2 or 3 hours.)

60 — Some growth of food poisoning bacteria may occur.

40 — Cold temperatures permit slow growth of some bacteria that cause spoilage.*

— Freezing temperatures stop growth of bacteria but may allow bacteria to survive. (Do not store food above 10° F. for more than a few weeks.)

*Don't store raw meats for more than 5 days or poultry, fish, or ground meat for more than 2 days in the refrigerator.

A final word: Alice

Because most poisoning victims are children, it's fitting that the best—and perhaps most famous—example of how to avoid a poisoning accident comes from a child, a 10-year-old girl named Alice. Many, many years ago, Alice was sitting on a riverbank listening to her sister read a book. The book was dull, the day was warm, and Alice's thoughts were already wandering when she happened to notice a large, well-dressed rabbit run by talking to himself. As curious as any child, Alice followed the rabbit. She soon found herself at the bottom of a very deep rabbit hole confronted by a bottle with a paper label tied around its neck. On the label were the words "Drink me."

Alice was facing a potential poisoning accident. Her next moves were very important:

> It was all very well to say "Drink me," but the wise little Alice was not going to do *that* in a hurry. "No, I'll look first," she said, "and see whether it's marked *'poison'* or not": for she had read several nice little stories about children who had got burnt, and eaten up by wild beasts, and other unpleasant things, all because they *would* not remember the simple rules their friends had taught them: such as, that a red-hot poker will burn you if you hold it too long; and that, if you cut your finger *very* deeply with a knife, it usually bleeds; and she had never forgotten that, if you drink much from a bottle marked "poison," it is almost certain to disagree with you, sooner or later.

The wise little girl is, of course, Alice from Lewis Carroll's *Alice's Adventures in Wonderland.* Her simple rules reflect the simpler world in which she lived. In our world, it isn't enough to check for the word *poison* when examining a strange bottle. We have our own simple rules, the rules we've covered in this book. Our rules may be different, but the example set by Alice is still correct: when faced with a potential poison, we should remember our simple rules—even if we find ourselves at the bottom of a rabbit hole. Children, in particular, must be taught rules that will help them avoid potential dangers. It was curiosity that led Alice down the rabbit hole, and all children are curious, a fact that should bring us nothing but joy.

Appendix 1: Common household poisons

Many products contain dangerous chemicals; so do most prescription and non-prescription medicines. The following is a list of the most common household poisons. This list isn't all-inclusive, and the contents of many products vary with the brand.

acetaminophen
acetone
acids
aerosols
airplane glue
alcohol
alcoholic beverages
ammonia
amphetamines
analgesics
aniline dyes
antidepressants
antifreeze (ethylene glycol)
antihistamines
antirust products
antiseptics
ant trap; ant syrup or paste
arsenic
aspirin
barbiturates
batteries (except dry cell)
benzene
bleaches
boric acid
brake fluid (for automobiles)
bromides
Campho-Phenique
camphor
carbon tetrachloride
carburetor cleaner (for automobiles)
chlorine bleach
cigarettes
cleaning fluids
Clinitest tablets
cold remedies
cologne
copper and brass cleaners
corn removers
cough medicines
cyanide
dandruff shampoo
denture cleansers
deodorizer cakes
deodorizers, room
detergents (dishwasher, laundry)
disinfectants
drain cleaners

dry-cleaning fluids
dyes
epoxy glue
epsom salts
fabric softeners
fertilizers
floor polishes and waxes
formaldehyde (including formalin)
furniture polishes and waxes
gas (natural)
gasoline
glue
gun cleaners
hair dyes, tints, colorings
herbicides
ink (indelible, laundry marking, and printer's)
insecticides
iodine
iron medications
kerosene
lacquers
laxatives
lighter fluid (cigarette, charcoal)
liniments
liquid naphtha
lye
Mercurochrome
mercury salts
Merthiolate
metal cleaners and polishes
methyl alcohol
methyl salicylate (oil of wintergreen)
model cement
moth balls
mouthwashes
muriatic acid
nail polish remover
nicotine
oil of wintergreen
oven cleaner
paint chips
paints (all types: acrylic, latex, lead base, oil base)
paint thinners and solvents
perfume

permanent wave solutions
peroxide
pesticides
petroleum distillates
phosphate-free detergents
pine oil
plant foods
polishes
prescription and nonprescription medicines
quicklime
rodenticides
rubbing alcohol
rug adhesives
rug cleaners
rust removers
sedatives
shaving lotion
shellacs
shoe dyes
shoe polishes
silver polish
sleep aids
soldering flux
spot removers
strychnine
sulfuric acid
suntan preparations
swimming pool chemicals
talc (talcum)
tobacco
toilet-bowl cleaner
tranquilizers
tricyclic antidepressants
turpentine
typewriter cleaners
varnishes
veterinary products
vitamins, fat soluble (A, D, E, K)
vitamins, with iron
wallpaper cleaners
wart removers
weed killers
window cleaners
windshield washer fluid (methyl alcohol)
witch hazel
wood preservatives

Appendix 2: Nontoxic substances

The following substances are considered nontoxic: they're harmful only in very large quantities. However, any substance can cause an unexpected reaction in certain individuals.

antacids
antibiotics
aquarium products
baby oil
ball-point inks (the amount in one pen)
bathtub toys (fluid-filled)
batteries, dry cell
birth-control pills
blackboard chalk
bubble bath
candles (insect-repellent type may be toxic)
caps for cap pistol
castor oil
crayons (children's: marked AP or CP or CS 130-146)
dehumidifying packets (silica or charcoal)
denture adhesives
deodorants
diaper rash ointment
eye makeup
fishbowl products
glycerin (glycerol)
graphite
gums (acacia, agar, ghatti)
hand creams and lotions
hormones
kaolin (Kaopectate)
lanolin

lauric acid
linoleic acid
linseed oil (not boiled)
lipstick
magnesium silicate (antacid)
makeup
matches
modeling clay
nail polish
paraffin, chlorinated
pencil lead (graphite)
petroleum jelly (petrolatum)
putty
red oil (turkey-red oil)
saccharin
sachets
shaving cream
silica
soaps (toilet bars)
spermaceti
stearic acid
sweetening agents
tallow
teething rings
thermometer fluid or mercury
toothpaste
toys, fluid filled
vitamins, multiple without iron
watercolor paints

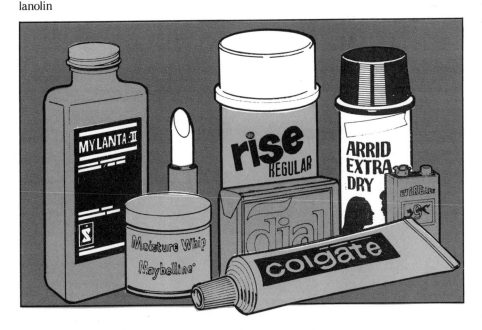

Appendix 3: Common poisonous plants

The following plants are poisonous in whole or in part:

Angel's-trumpet *(Datura suaveolens)*
Arrowhead *(Syngonium)*
Avocado *(Persea americana)*
Azalea *(Rhododendron)*
Bird-of-paradise flower *(Strelitzia reginae)*
Bittersweet, climbing nightshade, blue nightshade *(Solanum dulcamara)*
Black locust *(Robinia pseudoacacia)*
Black nightshade *(Solanum nigrum)*
Bleeding heart, Dutchman's-breeches *(Dicentra pussilla* and *D. cucullaria)*
Buttercup *(Ranunculus)*
Caladium *(Caladium)*
Candelabra cactus *(Euphorbia lactea)*
Castor bean *(Ricinus communis)*
Cherries, wild and cultivated *(Prunus)*
Christmas pepper *(Capsicum annum)*
Christmas rose, hellebore *(Helleborus niger)*
Coyotillo *(Karwinskia humboldtiana)*
Daffodil *(Narcissus)*
Daphne, spurge laurel *(Daphne mezereum)*
Deadly nightshade, belladonna *(Atropa belladonna)*
Delphinium *(Delphinium)*
Dumb cane, dieffenbachia *(Dieffenbachia)*
Elderberry, black and scarlet elders *(Sambucus canadensis* and *S. pubens)*
Elephant's ear, elephant ear *(Colocasia esculenta)*
Four-o'clock *(Mirabilis jalapa)*
Foxglove *(Digitalis purpurea)*
Golden chain *(Laburnum anagyroides)*
Holly *(Ilex)*
Hyacinth *(Hyacinthus orientalis)*
Hydrangea *(Hydrangea)*
Iris, blue flag *(Iris)*

Ivy, English, Boston, and others *(Hedera)*
Jack-in-the-pulpit *(Arisaema triphyllum)*
Jessamine, jasmine, yellow jessamine *(Gelsemium sempervirens)*
Jerusalem cherry *(Solanum pseudo-capsicum)*
Jimsonweed, thornapple, stinkweed *(Datura stramonium)*
Jonquil *(Narcissus jonquilla)*
Lantana, red sage, wild sage *(Lantana)*
Larkspur *(Delphinium ajacis)*
Laurel, mountain laurel, black laurel, sheep laurel, American laurel *(Kalmia)*
Lily of the valley *(Convallaria majalis)*
Marsh marigold, cowslip *(Caltha palustris)*
Mayapple *(Podophyllum peltatum)*
Mistletoe (American: *Phoradendron flavescens;* European: *Viscum album*)
Monkshood *(Aconitum)*
Moonseed *(Menispermum canadense)*
Morning glory, heavenly blue, pearly gates, flying saucers *(Ipomoea)*
Mother-in-law plant *(Dieffenbachia amoena)*
Narcissus *(Narcissus)*
Nutmeg *(Myristica fragrans)*
Oak *(Quercus)*
Oleander *(Nerium oleander)*
Philodendron *(Philodendron)*
Poison hemlock *(Conium maculatum)*
Pokeweed, pokeberry, scoke, inkberry *(Phytolacca americana)*
Pothos *(Scindapsus aureus; Rhaphidophora aurea)*
Privet, common privet *(Ligustrum vulgare)*
Rhododendron *(Rhododendron)*
Rosary pea or bean, jequirity bean, prayer bead, Indian licorice, crab's eye, precatory bean *(Abrus precatorius)*
Snow-on-the-mountain *(Euphorbia marginata)*
Star of Bethlehem *(Ornithogalum umbellatum)*
Sweet pea *(Lathyrus odoratus)*
Swiss cheese plant *(Monstera deliciosa)*
Tree tobacco *(Nicotiana glauca)*
Water hemlock, cowbane *(Cicuta)*
Wisteria *(Wisteria)*
Yew *(Taxus)*

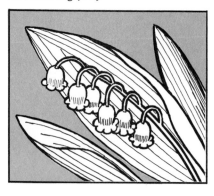

Appendix 4: Nonpoisonous plants

The following plants are considered nonpoisonous. Toxic symptoms from eating these plants are rare, but any plant can cause an unexpected reaction in certain people.

African violet *(Saintpaulia ionantha)*
Aluminum plant *(Pilea cadierei)*
Aspidistra, cast-iron plant *(Aspidistra)*
Aster *(Aster)*
Baby's tears *(Helxine soleirolii)*
Begonia *(Begonia)*
Bird's-nest fern *(Asplenium nidus)*
Boston fern *(Nephrolepis exaltata bostoniensis)*
Bougainvillaea *(Bougainvillaea)*
California poppy *(Eschscholtzia californica)*
Camellia *(Camellia)*
Christmas cactus *(Schlumbergera bridgesii, Zygocactus truncatus)*
Coleus *(Coleus blumei)*
Dahlia *(Dahlia)*
Dandelion *(Taraxacum officinale)*
Dracaena *(Dracaena)*
Easter lily, Bermuda lily *(Lilium longiflorum)*
Echeveria *(Echeveria)*
Gardenia *(Gardenia)*
Impatiens *(Impatiens)*
Jade plant *(Crassula argentea)*
Kalanchoe *(Kalanchoe)*
Lipstick plant *(Aeschynanthus lobbianus)*

Magnolia *(Magnolia)*
Marigold *(Tagetes)*
Moneywort, creeping Charlie, creeping Jennie *(Lysimachia nummularia)*
Nasturtium *(Tropaeolum)*
Norfolk Island pine *(Araucaria excelsa)*
Peperomia *(Peperomia caperata)*
Petunia *(Petunia)*
Poinsettia *(Euphorbia pulcherrima)*
Prayer plant *(Maranta)*
Purple passion *(Cynura aurantiaca)*
Rose *(Rosa)*
Sensitive plant *(Mimosa pudica)*
Snake plant, mother-in-law-tongue *(Sansevieria trifasciata)*
Spider plant *(Chlorophytum comosum)*
Swedish ivy *(Plectranthus australia)*
Tiger lily *(Lilium tigrinum)*
Umbrella tree *(Brassaia actinophylla* or *Schefflera actinophylla)*
Violet *(Viola)*
Wandering Jew *(Tradescantia fluminensis)*
Wax plant *(Hoya carnosa)*
Wild strawberry *(Fragaria)*
Zebra plant *(Aphelandra squarrosa)*

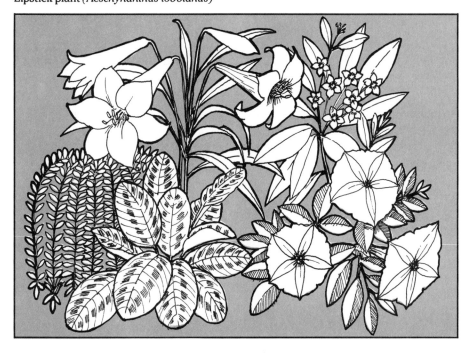

Index